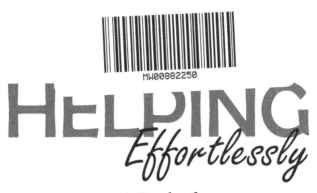

HELPING
Effortlessly

A Book of
Inspiration and Healing

Inspiring helpers because strong helpers
are the crux of strong communities

JENN BRUER

Helping Effortlessly
Copyright © 2018 by Jenn Bruer

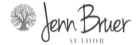

All rights reserved. No part of this publication
may be reproduced, distributed, or transmitted
in any form or by any means, including
photocopying, recording, or other electronic or
mechanical methods, without the prior written
permission of the author, except in the case of
brief quotations embodied in critical reviews and
certain other non-commercial uses permitted by
copyright law.

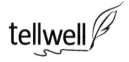

Tellwell Talent
www.tellwell.ca

ISBN
978-1-77370-860-7 (Paperback)
978-1-77370-859-1 (eBook)

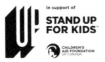

As a long-time foster parent, I am familiar with the barriers facing children and youth who have experienced abuse and neglect. I am passionate about improving the lives of young people and as a result, will donate 5% of the proceeds of each book sale to Stand Up for Kids.

Stand Up for Kids is Children's Aid Foundation of Canada's national campaign for child welfare, which aims to change the futures of Canada's most at-risk kids – those who have experienced abuse and neglect. We know that by helping these young people to overcome their trauma and break the cycle for future generations, they gain the strength and resilience to create a lifetime of their own unstoppable successes.

For more information on Stand Up for Kids and the Foundation's work, please visit cafdn.org

Dedication

This book is dedicated to my new friend, Kathy, and the countless other helpers I have met along my journey, people who have become a little broken because of child welfare, child protection, and their immeasurable contributions.

I hope this book is an inspiration to the helpers of the world to seek physical, emotional and spiritual healing, because the world needs you.

You ARE enough. You always have been. You always will be.

May this book be a small contribution to peace on earth.

Appreciation

I would like to express my deepest appreciation to those who helped make this book possible.

Firstly, I am grateful for my family, my wife Karen and my children: Sarah, Samuel, Sean, Ruth, Eden, and William. You mean the world to me.

A big thank-you to the editor of this book, Carola, you challenged me to be clearer, you tweaked words as though they were strokes on a canvas. I felt as if I was using crayons on a colouring page and after you came along it looked more like a painting.

A special acknowledgement to local Ontario artist Angela Lipscombe for providing your uplifting and inspirational artwork for the cover design.

I am grateful to the experts who assisted with formatting, cover design, and making this book look so great.

I want to thank the inspirational people along the way who seemingly showed up handing me bricks of knowledge and insight on how to heal: Dr Alan Christianson, Dr Terry Wahls, Robb Wolf, Dr. Natasha Campbell McBride, Chris Kresser, Dr. Sarah Ballantyne, Caroline Myss, his Holiness the 14th Dalai Lama, Desmond Tutu, and Eckhart Tolle. You may never know the impact you have had on me and on many others.

Lastly, to my wife, Karen, I could have accomplished none of this without your unwavering support. In this project, you encouraged and supported me, as you always do. I love you.

Table of Contents

SECTION 3: SPIRIT

Preface

Burnout (noun): - Exhaustion of physical or emotional strength or motivation, usually because of prolonged stress or frustration.

It can be a common belief that burnout is an inevitable consequence of being a lifelong helper, but does it have to be that way? While burnout obviously has something to do with stress, overdoing things, not being centred, and not listening to yourself or your body, one of the deepest contributors to burnout, I believe, is the deep disappointment of not living up to your true calling, which is to help.

As early as grade 5, I began to identify as a "helper," as someone who listened to other people's problems, someone who strived to make the world a better place. I had a deep yearning to uplift others, often children. As I grew and I saw people around me struggling, I became their counsellor. Whenever I could find the words and advice to inspire, uplift and effect positive change in the well-being of another, I turned to my true calling as a helper.

It's that journey that has brought me to where I am today, ready to share the things I have learned.

In 2011, I was 35 years old, a mother, foster parent, youth counsellor, wife and strong independent woman, among other things that were deeply important to me. But when I woke up one day feeling like a cliché, I knew I was burned out.

For many years leading up to that moment, I had made the mistake of thinking I was somehow immune to this phenomenon. Heck, we learn about burnout in school and it is a part of the language we use in helping fields. It's deeply woven into the helping culture as something we see everywhere but is rarely talked about or acknowledged when co-workers start to drop like flies from burnout.

So, while I knew what burnout was, I never thought it would happen to me. Even-keeled and rarely stressed out, I perhaps thought I was superwoman and nothing could break me. Burnout carries a stigma as a sign of weakness and since I am not weak, I think my young helper mind couldn't reconcile how burnout could come knocking at *my* door. But here I am, writing a book about how I faced and overcame my own burnout. Luckily for me (and maybe for you), burnout is not a character flaw.

But back to 2011… despite making most of my meals at home and being mostly vegetarian, I weighed 220 pounds. I had adult cystic acne – the kind that makes you not want to leave the house because it's embarrassing, itchy, and painful. I had mood swings, mild depression and felt like a sitting duck for a diagnosis of type 2 diabetes, which runs rampant in my family. Asthma, an affliction since babyhood, was severe and I was taking prescription preventative inhalers every day at the maximum dosage. My allergies were getting worse every year, requiring me to take prescription antihistamines even in winter. I broke out in hives for no apparent reason, my skin itched and my nose was permanently stuffed.

I was exhausted. And I needed to find a way to get healthy.

Fast forward to 2018 and the great news is, I healed. I am inspired, proud and excited to be on the other side of a transformation, and celebrating by writing this book.

I am sharing my story in the hope you'll come to believe that healing *is* possible. I will walk you through every intricate step of the very personal path I took, so that your path to healing can be a little easier. More important than believing healing is possible, I hope you reach the end of this book believing it is necessary.

Forcing myself to delve deep into how I transformed was cathartic for me, and I overcame a lot of resistance to get there. This book holds some of my deepest truths and life lessons; it is vulnerability in the most real sense. I worried about what I, a mum from the suburbs, could teach anyone else. But in the end, my mantra was these wise words from U.S. research professor Brené Brown:

> *"Failure can become our most powerful path to learning, if we're willing to choose courage over comfort."*

Writing *Helping Effortlessly* is my act of choosing courage over comfort.

This book is structured as a guide, and I hope you will read every sentence with an open heart. If something doesn't resonate or doesn't feel right for you, I hope you will adapt those parts according to what you DO believe and what IS right for you.

Eat your vegetables!

We hear this message a lot, and we don't doubt its truth. But let's be honest, most of us need a reminder because we probably don't eat enough veggies. We read diet books already knowing that avoiding sugar and eating more vegetables is a good place to start.

That is what I plan to do in this book – not "teach" you anything, but remind you of truths you probably already know. I'll ask questions because no transformation can truly happen without them.

Let's start with asking yourself this question:

Do I want peace on earth?

I am asking this question because, to truly contribute to peace, we have to want it. Ask this, then answer it with absolute vigour. There was a time in my life when I would have resisted answering this question because, with a heavy heart, I felt like it wasn't even possible. I am hopeful that you will keep trying to answer this question with love and truth. If you don't believe peace is possible, challenge yourself to keep asking this until, to your delight, you begin to believe it is possible.

Peace begins with me (and you).

Help (verb): Make it easier or possible for (someone) to do something by offering them one's services or resources.

> *"We can't help everyone, but everyone can help someone." – former U.S. president Ronald Reagan*

Being a helper can be unforgiving and a brutal undertaking. What does it mean to help?

In the context of this book I often refer to a "helper" in the professional sense: the people who spend their lives helping in various settings in the hopes of making the world a better place, people who see a need and feel they can contribute in some way. Those who are not helpers by profession still offer help; in fact, most people are helpers in some way or another.

While I often refer to "frontline workers" or people in social services who were involved in my experiences, I hope my story of healing and transformation will inspire all helpers. I want to take a moment to acknowledge the powerful and supportive people who help communities in so many ways and give selflessly of themselves. They are: the frontline worker who knows homeless people by name and ensures they have beds and blankets; the foster parent who takes in a child who has suffered unthinkable abuse; the social services worker who checks that the man down the street has taken his medication; the developmental service worker who helps the student in a wheelchair use the washroom; the concerned volunteer Big Brother to a boy who suffers from isolation; the child-and-youth worker who attends to the violent students in our schools; the frontline nurses, paramedics, police, teachers and many more important "helpers" who make our society run.

I have witnessed so many incredible, wonderful helpers slowly become broken by their job, their calling, their life's work.

This book is about how to be a better helper, how to inspire, uplift and effect positive change in others by first helping yourself. To be a better parent, a better social worker, foster parent, youth counsellor or better anything, you must first focus on YOU.

What does it mean to be a helper?

I contemplated what has helped me, and many of the greatest moments of inspiration have been in the moment I stood before a tree.

A tree helps me.

A tree makes me feel deeply grounded.

A tree transforms me; it reminds me of who I am.

A tree aligns me.

A well-choreographed dance

This book is divided into 3 sections because that is how my journey progressed.

Body

Mind

Spirit

Section 1: Body

"Take care of your body. It's the only place you have to live." – Entrepreneur and motivational speaker Jim Rohn

Epigenetics

Epigenetics (noun): Biology, the study of changes in organisms caused by modification of gene expression rather than alteration of the genetic code itself.

The body is wise, like a diary keeping details of our experiences. Stress can become trapped in our body, with signs reflected in every tiny cell that makes up the whole.

In an article entitled "Epigenetics: How to Alter Your Genes" in the U.K.'s The Telegraph, Chris Bell explains that epigenetics is a relatively new branch of genetics that has been declared the most important biological discovery since DNA. Until recently, it was believed you were stuck with the genes you were born with but now, thanks to epigenetics, it's known that your genes get turned on and off and are expressed to greater or lesser degrees depending on lifestyle factors.

And the book entitled *Super Genes* by Deepak Chopra and Rudolph Tanzi explains that only 5% of disease-related gene mutations are fully deterministic while 95% can be influenced by diet, behaviour and other environmental conditions.

Let that sink in: the influences of our lifestyle have control over our gene expression.

Gone are the days when we could blame it all on our genes. This is the reason to take heed and start making changes in body, mind and spirit. In the following chapters, I'll describe how I took back control over my body with the hopes of eventually controlling its biological expression.

> *"The word is out on the street that diet really does matter." – Clinical professor of medicine Dr. Terry Wahls*

Ask yourself these questions:

Am I afraid of changing my diet?

Is changing my diet a good idea?

Before I discuss diet, here are a few words of tough love and two tiny rants… please humour me!

Rant #1 – the art of confusion

People all around are using confusion as an excuse to continue eating the way they do. The fact is sugar and processed foods are addictive, and some people find facing this addiction so hard that they make excuses like "I don't where to begin," or "I didn't know that was a carbohydrate."

Letting confusion get in the way of changing your diet and lifestyle will deter you from facing the reality of how hard it is to give up sugar. If you'll forgive the expression, I am not going to sugar-coat it: sugary drinks, donuts, cake, cookies and candy are out. And there's no "okay in moderation."

What does that mean: once a week, once on the weekend, only on holidays? It probably doesn't mean Friday after work until Monday morning!

Rant # 2 – food fight

We seem to be looking for any excuse to fight. We have become so anchored to our ego that we use food and diet to engage in the stupidest "food fight" ever: the vegans/vegetarians versus the meat eaters.

Each of us wants to fuel our bodies and walk the earth with health and energy, to honour the vessel that takes us through life. We have allowed food, of all things, to divide us. Food is meant to bring us together. Food is celebratory, nourishing. Our world needs less conflict and more "live and let live."

Some of my dearest friends are vegetarian and I am a meat eater. While we have differing opinions and perspectives, we can still agree to disagree and love one another despite our differences. What is right for one may not be right for another and that is okay. We can be advocates for what we believe in with love and not anger.

This reminds me of a wonderful warrior who illustrates how to fight with love. Several years ago, a 19-year-old University of Iowa engineering student, Zach Wahls, stood up in the Iowa House of Representatives to deliver a speech about his life and experience growing up with two moms. His speech, available on YouTube, was a response to proposed legislative efforts to end civil unions in his state. In his advocacy address, Zach resonates love, not anger.

I must admit, I used to have the fantasy of being vegan. I felt like it would somehow make me cool, or as cool as you can be with developing crow's feet, stretch marks and a 14-yr-old son who, after hearing me sing in the car, says things like, "Oh my gawd, I think Mom just killed cool!"

But I digress … I somehow felt veganism would make me super-skinny and that I could have a really awesome (read "young and pretty") Instagram account where I would be wearing my Lululemon yoga pants and perfecting a downward dog while holding my Starbucks tall, bag-in green tea for my (thousands of) followers. I would be demonstrating the fun and glamour of meat avoidance because somehow, I would be ethically superior in all my glorious economic white privilege.

What's funny about that fantasy is it wasn't even mine. These imagery associations were unconsciously embedded in my brain, as ridiculous as I knew they were.

If you have found a diet that works, I am happy for you. As you move through this world advocating for what you believe in, do it with love and an open heart, not with anger and a closed heart.

End rants.

When I first started changing my diet, I gave up Diet Coke, which was a huge addiction for me. At first, I only had it when I went out for dinner, no more than once a month.

I can recall the last Diet Coke I had, believing aspartame to be a neurotoxin but knowing I was no longer addicted. I was proud of myself for practicing moderation yet felt an overwhelming conflict. It dawned on me how silly it was to be "practicing moderation" with a neurotoxin. It was like saying, "yeah, I used to snort cocaine every day but now I just do it when I go out for dinner. I am so healthy, I practice moderation and it is an incredible improvement."

I was no longer kidding myself.

Now I drink organic ginger kombucha and I have experienced firsthand that changes to food and diet can be a powerful tool towards healing the body. If you are living in a state of constant pain, you can change your diet and although it might not cure what ails you, it can help.

Many people feel angry by the idea of giving up sugar. If you are one of them, ask yourself this question:

What am I afraid of?

If you are afraid of putting in the work, I get that. You must get to a place where you think you are worth that amount of energy. Make yourself a priority.

Shortly after the realization that I had become a cliché case of burnout in 2011, I changed my diet to a "Paleo" diet, which dramatically altered my life; a fog that had plagued me for years was lifted.

That year I went from a size 20 to a size 10, but it wasn't just the weight that disappeared. I noticed lifelong phobias vanish, mild depression lift, mood swings become a thing of the past, cystic acne ... check! My morning stiffness was gone, and I felt emotionally and physically stronger in ways I never knew was possible.

Let me walk you through the Paleo diet, in simple and brief terms. If you want more information, a list of resources at the end of the book will point you in the right direction.

In layman's terms, Paleo means to eat like a caveman once did. It's only in the past 10,000 years that farming and agriculture was even a thing. According to the theory of

Paleo, we were not designed to eat grains, beans and legumes, especially in large quantities, if even at all, because in the natural caveman world, those foods would have been too labour-intensive and required too much processing to even be considered food.

If you really think about it, wheat requires a lot of processing to become digestible and yet we sometimes don't think of wheat foods as being highly processed. There is more to it than this, like the fact that some people believe that wheat causes systemic inflammation and other biological issues leading to the development of disease. Dr. William Davis, author of *Wheat Belly,* explains: "Grains also contain wheat germ agglutinin (WGA), a lectin protein in wheat. The lectin proteins of grains are, by design, nature's form of bodyguards. These toxins discourage molds, fungi, and insects from eating seeds of plants … I call wheat and its closely related grains not just perfect chronic poisons, but also perfect obesogens: foods that are perfectly crafted to make you fat, especially in the abdomen, what I call a wheat belly."

Since my eyes were opened to the Paleo diet, it has evolved to more of a science-based perspective with a following of highly respected, warrior-like people.

Here is the basic four-point plan that I began to follow in 2011:

1. DO EAT anything that could be hunted or gathered as we did in the caveman years: things like meats, fish, nuts, leafy greens, fruits, veggies, tubers and seeds.
2. DO EAT fermented foods such as kombucha, sauerkraut, kimchi, pickles and so on to restore and maintain healthy bacteria in the gut.

3. DON'T EAT pasta, cereal, sugar, beans, legumes, dairy and candy.
4. DON'T EAT anything that didn't exist in caveman times.

While most people don't follow Paleo religiously, the idea is to eat and drink what will help us be better, healthier versions of ourselves.

I have struggled with obesity from the age of 12, trying every diet you can think of: the cabbage soup diet (don't do it), vegetarianism, Canada's food guide (an absolute disgrace), Weight Watchers, Atkins, drinks, shakes, fasts. I am happy I found Paleo when I did, and I believe the crescendo of healing that followed may not have even have happened if not for the newfound energy and enlightenment that Paleo brought me.

Ask yourself this question:

Does food have the power to heal my body?

I felt so invigorated by my experience with this diet that I wanted to shout it from the roof tops: "Paleo can really change your life and your health!" I was meeting people who had adopted the Paleo lifestyle; some had been sick and improved their health conditions; some were cured from disease; some experienced weight loss; some experienced increased energy. But everyone I met in this community felt better.

I couldn't help but feel sad at the realization that our health-care system was continuing to tell us lies such as "low-fat diets are best" when, in fact, that was not what I and others were experiencing. I began to face the reality that our food and agriculture industries are in bed with our health-care industry, and that I needed to take control over my own health and disease prevention.

To share my message that food heals, I became a food coach. I held workshops, blogged and became a personal coach to people who wanted help with diet and health. I loved it but the Paleo perspective runs so counter to mainstream thinking that I could sense the skeptics around me. A friend even told me she was sick of seeing my Paleo posts on Facebook. Feeling like I wasn't doing a good job of spreading my message, I eventually stopped formally coaching.

A couple of years later though, I realized I had made an impact after all. People in my life and from my blog were reaching out to me for advice on health and diet. And then I read this life-changing quote:

> *"You don't know what a big act is, it's not for you to know." – Best-selling author and speaker Caroline Myss*

What did Caroline mean by this?

She tells a story of a man who, feeling great despair, decided that life was just too hard and he was going to end it that day. Walking home, as he decided on his suicide plan, he stopped at the corner near his apartment. A car pulled up and he waved the woman on as if to say, "No, you go ahead." She smiled at him and drove off.

That smile, that moment changed his life forever. Something about it gave him the will to survive. In that instant, he felt so touched by her grace that he decided to live. This is the story of how a woman's mere smile saved a man's life, and she may never know her incredible impact. It was not for her to know. We all make personal impacts but few of us will ever be aware of their depth.

As helpers, we often feel the need to see our impact in tangible, measurable ways. We allow negative language into our head about the "broken system;" we look through a lens of "it doesn't matter, I can't make a difference." But all together, we *can* make a difference even if we won't ever know it.

A few years ago, I fostered a 12-year-old girl. She was challenging and rarely happy with what we said or provided. She always seemed angry and it seemed like we never made an impact. (It's common for foster parents to look for behavioural changes and stabilization as proof of a job well done.) After a short placement, this young girl moved. I saw her a year later and she looked like a new person. When I said with surprise, "What happened to you?", she said, "You happened to me!"

Sometimes we see the impact and sometimes we don't. It is not always for us to know.

Luckily, I managed to heal my body before disease set in and that is something for which I am so grateful.

One of my mentors is Dr. Terry Wahls. I urge you to read her story if you are looking for more inspiration about the healing powers of food – she has an amazing TED Talk. Terry went from using a tilt and recline wheelchair due to progressive multiple sclerosis to participating in bike marathons six months after changing her diet. No question, the Paleo lifestyle truly changed me, but it's not the only way to heal through diet. Others have found different guidelines that have helped them heal.

I have also found *The Food Babe* by Vani Hari very inspiring; she is taking on the food industry fight on our behalf. She lobbies to have toxic ingredients removed from our food supply, calling out the food manufacturers and distributors on substances like aspartame that are proven to be bad for us. The following article from a medical journal is entitled "Increasing Brain Tumor Rates: Is there a link to aspartame?" "Compared to other environmental factors putatively linked to brain tumors, the artificial sweetener aspartame is a promising candidate to explain the recent increase in incidence and degree of malignancy of brain tumors. Evidence potentially implicating aspartame includes an early animal study revealing an exceedingly high incidence of brain tumors in aspartame-fed rats compared to no brain tumors in concurrent controls, the recent finding that the aspartame molecule has mutagenic potential, and the close temporal association (aspartame was introduced into US food and beverage markets several years prior to the sharp increase in brain tumor incidence and malignancy). We conclude that there is need for reassessing the carcinogenic potential of aspartame."

I can't even say aspartame without cringing; we were told this was an acceptable alternative to sugar, but they lied or were wrong. Either way, we were misled. They said aspartame was going to help us get skinny but we now know this isn't true since several large-scale prospective cohort studies found positive correlation between artificial sweetener use and weight gain.

Pediatric endocrinologist Dr. Robert Lustig has some great information on this in his life-changing lecture, "Sugar: The Bitter Truth," on YouTube.

I simplify this whole aspartame argument like this: if it's generated in a lab, it's probably not a good thing for me to consume. Period. Previously, I would have been completely oblivious to the safety of aspartame, blindly consuming it with the assumption that my government had my back. But look around and you can see signs of consciousness emerging.

Now, after the help of some truly inspirational leaders in the health community, I simply focus on eating real food, as if I were a caveman but with hydro, running water – and a Vitamix blender! I do occasionally eat rice, a little dairy, xylitol and stevia, all of which are most certainly not Paleo, but here is the difference: I eat those foods as treats, and not under the false pretense that they're healthy for me. Mostly, I try to stick to good quality fresh meats (pasture-raised and ethically treated) and large portions of vegetables emphasizing leafy greens.

If you have avoided diet changes, it could be because you are overwhelmed. In that case, I suggest beginning by just changing your breakfast habits. Consider looking at food differently, as a source of fuel and nutrition instead of something fast, easy or cheap to obtain. I love the hashtag #JERF which is "Just Eat Real Food." So many so-called diets can be daunting and the science confusing, with conflicting messages thrown around depending on whose agenda is attached to them. I urge you not to engage in that confusion. Instead, think of REAL food as food that is found on the earth and hasn't been heavily processed. Even pasta and breads have been to a manufacturer. Crackers are not whole foods. Think about what makes your body feel good, not what makes you feel like you belong to some diet group. If avoiding meat gives you more energy, then do that. Just do you.

Repeat after me:

Food has the power to heal my body.

Before I close the discussion on diet, I want to note that while I have had such great healing success following a Paleo food guide, I do ensure that I consume a healthy amount of carbohydrates. Often people in the Paleo community advocate for a more ketogenic approach, keeping carbohydrate intake below 50 grams and at times even below 20 grams per day. But you can eat high carbs or low carbs on a Paleo diet, it's up to you. I have found that I fare best with a carbohydrate intake of 90 to 120 grams (net carbohydrates after the deduction of fibre grams). I try to get my carbohydrates from complex carbs like sweet potato. I learned about the importance of carbohydrates on burnout recovery from a book called *The Adrenal Reset Diet* by Dr. Alan Christianson. I highly recommend this as a resource for burnout recovery; much of the information in this section of my book I owe to his expertise.

> *"I've seen so many people who when they've gone on a low carb, their sugar gets higher and they have higher levels of cortisol because the body is overcompensating." – Dr. Alan Christianson*

Ask your BODY these questions:

What foods make my body feel healthy?

What kinds of foods make my body feel sluggish?

What does my body want me to change?

Light therapy & sleep

Ask yourself this question:

Does light affect me?

The studies on sleep are exploding; we know how important it is to our mental and our physical health.

In a study led by endocrinology expert Eve Van Cauter, PhD, healthy men and women with an average body mass index were tested for hormonal changes after sleep deprivation. Half of the subjects were normal sleepers, the other half averaged 6 ½ hours or less. Glucose tolerance tests showed that the short sleepers experienced hormonal changes that could affect their future body weight and impair their long-term health, the National Sleep Foundation reported. To keep their blood sugar levels normal, the short sleepers needed to make 30% more insulin than the normal sleepers. Cauter called sleep deprivation "the royal route to obesity." Despite not yet being overweight, "these young adults had profiles that predisposed them to putting on weight," she concluded.

In my journey towards healing from burnout, I needed to address many factors to encourage my body to perform optimally. As someone with lifelong insomnia and sub-optimal sleep performance, I knew that in addition to diet, I needed to fix my sleep. But how?

This led me to the question: Do we need sunlight? Experts have been warning us about the dangers of over-exposure to the sun's UV rays and the risk of skin cancer, but new research is pointing us in another direction, suggesting that too little sunlight can be equally harmful to our health.

In an article entitled "Benefits of Sunlight: A Bright Spot for Human Health," published in the Environmental Health Perspectives, US National Library of Medicine, the World Health Organization (WHO) conducted studies highlighting the fact that our need for light might be far greater than our need to protect ourselves from the sun. The studies also determined that insufficient exposure to light has far greater consequences than too much light and looked at how insufficient light exposure contributes to the symptoms of adrenal fatigue.

At the core of our health in many ways is full spectrum lighting and the natural light we receive from sunlight. Like many others, my life had become so off-kilter and out of sync with nature that I was unintentionally robbing myself of the vital energy that sunlight provides.

Our circadian rhythm cycles follow an approximate 24-hour pattern, responding to light and dark. Circadian rhythms determine a whole host of functions including sleep-to-wake cycles and body temperature. If these rhythms get disrupted, a range of issues can arise, from sleep disorders to depression and weight gain. In an article entitled "Circadian Rhythm," published by the National Institute of General Medical Sciences, it is confirmed that light has a profound effect on natural circadian rhythms. Contributing factors to sleep disruption include shift work, exposure to light that is out of sync with nature and artificial indoor lighting.

During the winter months, especially here in Canada, getting enough exposure to sunlight can be challenging if not impossible. Waking up in the dark and coming home from work in the dark makes it tough. Let's talk about some strategies on how to re-boot the natural body clock without having to freeze our buns off outside.

Before the dawn of electricity, the most powerful signal to our circadian rhythm was the bright light of the rising sun and the orange glow of the fire that we would gather around after sunset. These distinct changes in the levels of light were signals to the body to reduce sleep hormones like melatonin and increase the awake hormones like cortisol.

Ideally if we get our light intake from the sun we benefit not only from the factors mentioned but from vitamin D. The research, which is exploding, shows there is no question about the importance of vitamin D to our optimal health.

Most people don't rise and sleep with the sun anymore. But modern technology in the form of full spectrum lighting and dawn simulator alarm clocks can help reset this pattern. While they may be expensive, these products can have real and lasting benefits in repairing circadian rhythms.

Dawn simulator alarm clocks

One of my best investments was a dawn simulator alarm clock, fitted with small lamps that gradually brighten to mimic the effects of a natural sunrise. My alarm clock also has a fun feature of chirping birds to wake you – although I often hear the real thing and wonder if I need to turn off the alarm. For the product to really work, it's important to buy an alarm with a high light intensity.

Full spectrum lighting box

Along the same lines is the full spectrum lighting box. The greatest benefit will come with lights that emit at least 10,000 lux (measure of light intensity). I find that at least thirty minutes of exposure within an hour of waking seems to really keep my rhythm on target.

Blue light blockers

The short-wave blue light emitted from our screened devices can affect the body's ability to produce melatonin. We all know that looking at a screen right before bed can cause harm to our rhythm but there are tools that can help.

The best solution is to avoid looking at any phone, computer or TV screen in the hour before going to sleep. But abstinence isn't always easy and if you're like me and you like to (shamefully) play "Candy Crush" before bed, then here are a few options:

- Install a program called *L-Lux* which adjusts the device's colour display according to the time of day.
- Install low-wattage (under 40 watts) orange-coloured light bulbs in your bedroom. (Amber lights tell our body it's time to sleep.)
- Purchase a blue-light blocking screen protector for your devices to protect eyes from the blue light being emitted.

One of the best quality reading lights for maintaining a healthy circadian rhythm – I have one for my children too – is the SomniLight brand. They have a variety of other light therapy products as well.

The most unsexy glasses ever

This is the least sexy option but it's the one I like the best. The Blue Blocking Glasses by Uvex I purchased are orange-tinted and block almost all blue light from all sources. They are safety glasses too, which contributes to their appearance as the most unsexy glasses ever.

Blue light is in the overhead lights in our bedrooms and all around our home so placing a cover over my phone might protect me from that blue light but not from other sources before bed. So I wear my unsexy glasses an hour before bed to protect me from all sources and to signal my body to stop producing cortisol, to start producing melatonin, and to get ready for deep slumber.

Adaptogen (noun): Any of various natural substances used in herbal medicine to normalize and regulate the systems of the body.

Ask yourself this question:

Can herbs and supplements help me?

The adrenal glands reside just above the kidneys and help our body regulate blood pressure, metabolism and electrolytes. They produce hormones for dealing with stress and cortisol regulation in the body. From a biological perspective, when you perform as a helper, the adrenal glands take a beating. If you handle stress well, it's thanks to the help from your adrenal glands. Therefore, supporting your adrenal function should be a part of preventing or treating burnout.

Adrenal supplements, which help support adrenal glands, have been a phenomenal tool in my path toward health. You may hear the term "adrenal fatigue" being thrown around in the natural-health community, although some argue it's not a thing. But being drained and stressed *is* a thing and should be addressed, particularly in helpers.

In the face of burnout there are natural herbs and substances called adaptogens that can help support our body, adrenals and energy levels. As always, ensure your doctor is on board with any changes in your health regime including the use of adaptogens. Here are a few examples:

Tulsi Tea

Tulsi Tea (ocimum sanctum), sometimes referred to as "holy basil," is a potent herb that has been used in India for thousands of years. Tulsi, a shrub that grows to about 18 inches, has leaves that are oval and serrated, with colours ranging from light green to dark purple. They offer a rich source of essential oil and flavonoids. Tulsi contains antioxidant and anti-depression properties that help reduce the damaging effects of stress and aging on the body.

According to a study by Ayurveda Integrative Medicine, while modern scientific research suggests that tulsi is effective in treating a range of stressful conditions, within Ayurveda, tulsi is more commonly recommended for enhancing the ability to adapt to psychological and physical stress, and therefore prevent the development of stress-related diseases. To this end, many Ayurvedic practitioners recommend the regular consumption of tulsi tea as an essential lifestyle practice.

Lemon Balm Tea

Used since ancient times to calm the heart and the body, lemon balm, with its delicate lemony flavour, lifts the spirit and any culinary dish to which it is added. It has been used to sweeten jam and jellies, as an addition to salad, and as a flavouring for fish and poultry dishes, and liqueurs. Lemon balm is also used as an ingredient in perfumes, cosmetics and furniture polish. It's often found as a tea in combination with other relaxing herbs such as valerian, as well as an essential oil and in topical ointments.

Licorice root

Licorice root supplements can give the adrenal gland some relief by stimulating it and promoting a healthy level of cortisol in the body. For that reason, it's best to take this root earlier in the day.

Sometimes when the adrenals become taxed, low blood pressure develops. When this happened to me, I found licorice root to be a life saver because it increased blood pressure.

For that reason, you should avoid taking licorice root if you have high blood pressure. People who are sensitive to licorice should also proceed with caution.

Ashwagandha

Ashwagandha, sometimes referred to as Indian ginseng, is said to be one of the most powerful herbs in Ayurvedic healing. This powerful root is known to relieve anxiety and help regulate the immune system. Research has shown noticeable results in lowering levels of cortisol and balancing thyroid hormones. Some benefits include mood improvement, support for brain health, increased sex drive, menopausal support and memory boost.

According to a study published on PubMed US National Library of Medicine in 2012, menopausal women who took ashwagandha found a reduction in symptoms like irritability, anxiety and hot flashes. Multiple studies have discovered one of the primary reasons that ashwagandha is so effective at supporting brain health is that it contains antioxidants that can destroy the free radicals that lead to premature aging.

Rhodiola

In 2009 a scientist in Sweden conducted a trial testing rhodiola's impact on people suffering with stress-related fatigue. They found rhodiola has an anti-fatigue effect that increases mental performance – particularly the ability to concentrate – and decreases cortisol response to awakening stress in burnout patients with fatigue syndrome.

Maca root

Maca root (Lepidium meyenii) is known for its ability to enhance fertility, as an aphrodisiac, and for its beneficial effects on energy, mood and blood pressure, among other health issues. Maca is a cruciferous vegetable native to the Andes mountains of Peru. It looks like a radish or turnip, and is consumed both as a dietary staple and medicinal herb. The main edible part of maca is the root, which grows underground. Maca is a broad-based food that in many cases can support and rejuvenate overwhelmed, tired adrenal glands and other aspects of the hormonal system. Over time, use of maca can lead to greater energy, stamina, clarity of mind and spirit, and the ability to handle stress.

Go easy on the stimulants

One more piece of advice on taking care of your adrenals: go easy on the stimulants, especially ubiquitous caffeine. Diet

Coke, regular Coke, caffeinated drinks, coffee and energy drinks. Avoid these as much as you can, preferably limited to one in the morning, or ditch them all together.

Stimulants push the adrenal glands to produce more cortisol, which is why we reach for them. The more you push with stimulants, the more exhausted the adrenals can become.

Vitamin D

Vitamin D plays a crucial part in balancing stress in the body and helping overcome the effects of stress. Since adrenal fatigue can be a result of chronic and prolonged stress, fatigue and lethargy are the most common symptoms of this condition but they can also include hair loss, weight gain, sleep disturbance and other signs. With Seasonal Affective Disorder (SAD), neurotransmitter imbalance can also be a common symptom.

Vitamin D has immune-boosting effects and optimal levels of vitamin D can help encourage the body to regulate stress. For adrenal health and overall health, recent research makes it clear that it's truly important to get your vitamin D.

Health Canada recommends supplementation of vitamin D, according to the following chart on their website.

Age group	Recommended Dietary Allowance (RDA) per day	Tolerable Upper Intake Level (UL) per day
Infants 0-6 months	200 mg (*)	1000 mg
Infants 7-12 months	260 mg (*)	1500 mg
Children 1-3 years	700 mg	2500 mg
Children 4-8 years	1000 mg	2500 mg
Children 9-18 years	1300 mg	3000 mg
Adults 19-50 years	1000 mg	2500 mg
Adults 51-70 years Men Women	1000 mg 1200 mg	2000 mg 2000 mg
Adults > 70 years	1200 mg	2000 mg
Pregnancy & Lactation 14-18 years 19-50 years	1300 mg 1000 mg	3000 mg 2500 mg

(*) Adequate Intake rather than Recommended Dietary Allowance.

When I was at my most stressed, I had my vitamin D levels tested, which showed a deficiency. Based on anecdotal experience, my need for Vitamin D seems to increase during high levels of stress. I recommend testing first and then supplement accordingly. I test twice per year to ensure I am maintaining optimal levels.

I like to order tests online from a site called GrassrootsHealth.com and if you want to know more, I highly recommend their website for handy charts, recommendations on safe dosing, etc. Here is a little information on what they do, taken from their website:

"GrassrootsHealth is a nonprofit public health research organization dedicated to moving public health messages regarding vitamin D from research into practice. It has a panel of 48 senior vitamin D researchers from around the world contributing to its operations. GrassrootsHealth is currently running the D*action field trial to solve the vitamin D deficiency epidemic worldwide. Under the D*action umbrella, there are also targeted programs for breast cancer prevention and a 'Protect Our Children NOW!' program to stop vitamin D deficiency where it starts, in utero. In 2007, as Carole was recovering from breast cancer treatment, she stumbled upon a web site which touted vitamin D levels as being important, even preventive, for breast cancer. After more research she found that indeed this research was REAL. Why had she never heard it before? Could she have prevented her breast cancer? She started by garnering the support of many vitamin D researchers and GrassrootsHealth was born – with the mission of moving those researchers' findings into practice!"

GABA deficiency

GABA, short for gamma-aminobutyric acid, is a naturally occurring neurotransmitter that is used to relax the brain. I became of aware of my GABA deficiency through testing from my naturopath, and realized it was a contributing factor to my symptoms of burnout and adrenal fatigue.

Dr. Michael Lam wrote a detailed article online about GABA entitled "The Facts About GABA and Your Health." Here's a short excerpt: "These days, in everyday modern life, the sympathetic nervous system might be triggered on your commute to work, after a fight with a co-worker or partner, or another event that might make you angry and stressed. If left unchecked, your body would be under constant stress, so there must be a way to counteract this stress response … Reactions to stress, and activation of the sympathetic nervous system give you feelings of anxiety, fear, restlessness and the inability to fall asleep because of racing thoughts and "what if's". When active and functioning correctly, GABA is released to deactivate or inhibit these effects. GABA is referred to as **an inhibitory neurotransmitter**, because it turns these functions of the brain off temporarily. Epinephrine and nor-epinephrine are referred to as excitatory neurotransmitters because they turn functions of the brain on in situations of stress. GABA alleviates some of the anxiety and related symptoms associated with Adrenal Fatigue in advanced stages when the flight or fight response is activated. The mind and body connection make GABA very important while recovering from Adrenal Fatigue. GABA helps the body stay at rest and prevents your body from having a strong reaction to external stress. Below we will go into detail about how this works and how GABA is beneficial during Adrenal Fatigue recovery. As Adrenal Fatigue progresses into the later stages, cortisol levels eventually fall because the body can't produce enough cortisol to meet the demand and stress levels remain high in the body. The autonomic nervous system continues to release epinephrine and norepinephrine under the stress response. Your body tries to produce enough GABA to compensate, but levels become erratic. These erratic levels make balancing the hormones involved in the flight or fight response difficult, leading to the array of anxiety, restlessness, and feeling wired. Such experience during Adrenal Fatigue is the result of the neuro-affective response system as it becomes dysregulated."

I began to take GABA at night and, combined with my other sleep hygiene routines – exposure to full spectrum lighting in the morning, blue-blocking sun glasses at night, meditation, salt baths in the evenings – my sleep problem slowly resolved itself.

You don't necessarily need to test for GABA deficiency, you can simply try GABA supplements, with permission from your doctor, to see if you get any benefits. If you are suffering the effects of burnout there is a good chance you may be deficient in this amazing neurotransmitter.

Supplements I take

- Magnesium (600 mg of magnesium citrate per day)
- Vitamin K2 (100 mcg a day)
- Vitamin D (5000 IU in winter and 2000 IU in summer)
- Vitamin C (3000 mg per day)

- Omega 3 (1000 mg of omega 3 per day, increased if I have any signs of inflammation like stiff joints)
- Probiotics (one strong probiotic each day; favourite brand is Renew Life-Ultimate Flora)
- Adaptogens, as mentioned in this chapter (I rotate them every 2 months)
- GABA (500 mg at night)

Other supplements

Other supplements to consider if you struggle with mood-related issues include 5-HTP, L-theanine and taurine, all of which I have taken at one time or another with great success. None of these should be taken while on antidepressants, and it's essential to check with your doctor before experimenting with supplements of any kind.

Exercise

Ask yourself these questions:

Can exercise help me?

What exercise is right for me?

In the case of burnout/adrenal fatigue, exercise, especially in the form of cardio activity, can make the symptoms worse. In the book, *The Adrenal Reset Diet,* Dr. Alan Christianson writes: "**Prolonged and frequent high-intensity aerobic exercise will only make things worse**. Anything above half your maximum effort will cause substantial elevations in cortisol levels. Therefore, this will block fat loss, even though you might be burning more calories."

The exercises that have served me best in my burnout recovery are:

- Walking
- Hiking in nature
- Heavy lifting for short periods of time (for me 30 minutes of heavy lifting is perfect)
- Yoga

- Biking long distance, lower intensity, if I have the energy

Here in Ontario we had a horrid winter in 2017-2018 and the spring was a bitch too. The thaw never seemed to come and when it did Mother Nature sent a severe ice storm just as most of us were getting our winter tires off and putting the kids' snow pants away. And then we had a severe wind storm. I was driving in the storm with tears flowing down my face and screaming, "I don't want to die!"

But finally, spring-like weather presented itself complete with budding flowers and a warm breeze. I went for a hike with my wife along the Credit River in Mississauga, Ontario, and it was incredible. I obsessed about getting my steps in until halfway through when I felt myself getting tired. In the past I would have pushed myself harder, but that day I slowed down and I listened to my body.

Listen. Use exercise to uplift you and don't use it to push your body towards things that are not good for you or to prove you are a hard worker. Exercise until it feels good; if it feels bad, keep going but slow down. But don't sit on the couch all day.

The biggest shift for me in the way of exercise has been avoiding sitting for long periods of time. Since the average adult spends 50 to 70% of their time sitting, chances are likely that you are sitting as you read this. Chances are also high that you were sitting for the 60 minutes *before* reading this, and that you will probably sit for much of your day after reading.

We sit to eat breakfast. We sit in our cars en route to various destinations. We sit at our desks all day and then on the couch at night. Then guilt races through our heads as we think we probably should have gone to the gym to offset all that sitting.

And the worst part is, you have probably already heard that sitting is killing you.

If you are on social media, then you've most likely come across the newest headline "Sitting Is the New Smoking." This sensationalistic phrase was coined by Dr. James Levine, Director of the Mayo Clinic at Arizona State University, and it's seemingly everywhere. Countless studies have pointed to a correlation between chronic sitting and an increased risk for type 2 diabetes, cardiovascular disease, breast cancer and kidney disease in women, as well as numerous other chronic issues related to obesity and even death. According to Dr. Levine, "sitting is more dangerous than smoking, kills more people than HIV and is more treacherous than parachuting."

Essentially, we are sitting ourselves to death.

Many people and companies are finally taking heed and embracing the idea that standing desks can promote better health. But the problem is that regardless of whether you are sitting or standing, being in the same position with little or no movement for 60 to 90 minutes or more at a time is not healthy, so even if you set aside extra time to jog, bike, run or swim, you still aren't offsetting the negative effects of being sedentary for the vast majority of your day.

I am not suggesting that exercise is not a good idea – we should all be doing more of it – but we can no longer use the excuse that sitting for several hours a day is safe because we exercised for an hour.

According to bio mechanist Katy Bowman, author of *Move Your DNA*, you may actually be increasing your risk for cardiac problems by sitting all day then cramming in a workout at night. You may end up doing more harm than good. Luckily, I saved the best news for last in this study headed "Minimal Intensity Physical Activity (Standing and Walking) of Longer Duration Improves Insulin Action and Plasma Lipids More than Shorter Periods of Moderate to Vigorous Exercise (Cycling) in Sedentary Subjects When Energy Expenditure Is Comparable." Researchers suggest that simply reducing inactivity by increasing the time spent walking or standing is a more effective way to help reduce certain health risks than one hour of physical exercise.

So, what is the take-home message? We no longer must buy into an old-school "all or nothing" approach. Most of us have joined the gym and begun an intense exercise program only to drop off the following week because it was too much. Baby steps are okay, and often more effective.

When tackling your fitness goals, aim to be less sedentary. Just move more!

Try these simple tricks:

- ☐ Wherever you drive, park your car at the far end of the parking lot.
- ☐ Get a fitness tracker and try to increase your steps by 500 each day.
- ☐ Take the stairs instead of the elevator.
- ☐ At the office, walk to speak to your colleagues instead of emailing.
- ☐ Do squats while on the phone.
- ☐ Walk on the treadmill on long phone calls.
- ☐ Step away from your desk every hour for a 5-minute stretch and walk.

☐ Google 5-minute yoga stretches (you DO have 5 minutes).

The take home message is that reducing inactivity by increasing the time spent moving is a more effective way to help reduce certain health risks than a one-hour session of physical exercise.

Steps to reduce toxic load

Ask yourself this question:

Are there cosmetics or products in my life that could be toxic to me?

According to the World Health Organization's (WHO) February 2018 Cancer Fact Sheet, cancer is one of the leading causes of morbidity and mortality worldwide, with approximately 14 million new cases in 2012 (1), and the number of new cases expected to rise by about 70% over the next two decades.

Let that sink in: cancer is expected to rise by 70%. Most of us have already been touched by cancer. I think it's clear that we should all take heed. When discussing healing our body from a holistic perspective, it stands to reason that reducing our overall toxic load is a good idea in preventing cancer.

According to the nonprofit organization Environmental Working Group (EWG), the average newborn baby has almost 300 known toxins in his or her umbilical cord blood. That's just as a newborn – imagine the amount of toxins we are exposed to over a lifetime.

While diet and exercise clearly play a vital role in cancer prevention, there are other strategies we can use to reduce our exposure to toxic load. There are thousands of industrial chemicals on the market today. Not all of them have been tested as safe when it comes to influencing our health, especially over time.

Individuals (like me) who are determined to act for the prevention of cancer have taken matters into their own hands. By far the greatest resource that has helped me has been the Environmental Working Group. If you haven't heard of the EWG, here is a little about them taken from their website: "The Environmental Working Group's mission is to empower people to live healthier lives in a healthier environment. With breakthrough research and education, we drive consumer choice and civic action. We are a non-profit, non-partisan organization dedicated to protecting human health and the environment. We work for you. Do you know what's in your tap water? What about your shampoo? What's lurking in the cleaners underneath your sink? What pesticides are on your food? How about the farms, fracking wells and factories in your local area? Do you know what safeguards they use to protect your water, soil, air and your kids? Which large agribusinesses get your tax dollars and why? What are GMOs? What do they do to our land and water? More than two decades ago EWG set out to answer these questions, and more, and to empower you to get to know your environment and protect your health. EWG's groundbreaking research has changed the debate over environmental health. From households to Capitol Hill, EWG's team of scientists, policy experts, lawyers, communication experts and programmers has worked tirelessly to make sure someone is standing up for public health when government and industry won't. Through our reports, online databases, mobile apps and communications campaigns, EWG is educating and empowering consumers to make safer and more informed decisions about the products they buy and the companies they support. In response to consumer pressure, companies are giving up potentially dangerous chemical ingredients in their products and improving their practices."

Choosing organic food

The EWG has put a lot of work into providing the public with tips and tricks to reducing toxic load. They have compiled two lists to help customers reduce pesticides in produce. The first list is conveniently called "The Dirty Dozen," and the EWG recommends you always choose organic. The second list is called "The Clean Fifteen" but the EWG suggests it is not as necessary to purchase organic since they have little to no traces of pesticide residue and are safe to consume conventionally.

	The Dirty Dozen	The Clean Fifteen
1	Strawberries	Sweet Corn
2	Spinach	Avocadoes
3	Nectarines	Pineapple
4	Apples	Cabbage
5	Peaches	Onions
6	Pears	Sweet Peas
7	Cherries	Papaya

8	Grapes	Asparagus
9	Celery	Mangoes
10	Tomatoes	Eggplants
11	Sweet Bell Pepper	Honeydew
12	Potatoes	Kiwi
13		Cantaloupe
14		Cauliflower
15		Grapefruit

The EWG recommends choosing five servings of fruits and vegetables daily from the Clean Fifteen list to lower the volume and type of pesticides consumed by 92 %. For the full list of the 49 types of produce that the EWG tested and rated, you can visit their website at www.foodnews.org.

Hygiene products

Did it ever occur to you that some of the products we use every day like lotions, hair products, sunscreen and makeup all contain chemicals? It may surprise you to learn about the potentially harmful chemicals that companies sneak into these products, especially under the guise of "natural."

According to the EWG, chemicals found in hygiene and beauty products contain carcinogens, reproductive toxicants, common allergens, immune disrupting chemicals and more.

I like to review the products I use daily on the EWG database called "Skin Deep" – it's super user-friendly. They rate each product with a red, yellow or green light. I am not 100% about the products I choose but I certainly like to reduce the artificial fragrances. We tend to falsely believe that clean has a smell but this is not true. Dirty has a bad odour but clean has no odour. Your clean clothes should smell like cotton with an absence of bad odour, not like green apples that were created in a lab. These fragrances are all toxic; we breathe them in and then our bodies must get rid of those toxic substances. If you like nice smells, reach for organic essential oils instead of fragrances filled with products like laundry detergents, perfumes and soaps which are often filled with toxins.

Non-toxic cleaners

For many years I have been using a cleaning product called Pink Solution, which comes from a Canadian-owned and operated company, is naturally derived, eco-friendly and has no fragrance. It's also very inexpensive. There are plenty of eco-friendly cleaning products on the market but you can also consider using vinegar and water with microfibre cloths which is effective too.

House plants for cleaner indoor air quality

Given that we spend more time indoors than out, air quality matters. Poorly ventilated spaces and volatile substances found indoors all contribute to poor air quality and pollution indoors, but what can we do about it?

According to a report entitled "A study of interior landscape plants for indoor air pollution abatement" on the NASA Clean Air Study, it was confirmed that some common indoor plants have the remarkable ability to remove toxic compounds such as carcinogens, solvents and airborne pollutants from the air. From this study, NASA compiled a list of air-filtering plants that could help keep air clean in space station settings. Plants not only absorb carbon dioxide, they also release oxygen.

The research seems to suggest having a houseplant for every 100 square feet of indoor space. For my 3,000-square foot home that means 30 plants. I do have 20 so I'm getting close. House plants are also beautiful and improve the "Zen" of your space. Here are the top five houseplants that can improve your home's air quality and remove pollutants, according to the NASA study:

Peace lily

The peace lily tops the list in the air-cleaning department. They enjoy shady areas and moist soil, although mine reside in a full-sun spot in my kitchen and have quadrupled in size in 10 years. These plants bloom throughout the summer which can contribute some pollen and floral scents, but the blooms are gorgeous. Pollutants removed are ammonia, benzene, formaldehyde and trichloroethylene.

Spider plants

This is one of the easiest plants to take care of. If you forget to water it, it usually survives, and it's non-toxic to pets and children. They love bright, indirect sunlight and can grow in any soil. Pollutants removed are formaldehyde and xylene.

Snake plant/mother-in-law's tongue

Not only does this plant have the coolest name, it's also one of the hardest houseplants to kill as long as you don't overwater it. The snake plant prefers drier conditions and some indirect sunlight, although I have one in my front hall with very little sun and it thrives. Pollutants removed are formaldehyde, trichloroethylene, and benzene.

Aloe vera

Easy to grow, the aloe vera plant prefers dry conditions. I love aloe, which has well-known benefits. The gel inside the stalks is filled with clear liquid that contains vitamins, enzymes and amino acids that have wound-healing, antibacterial and anti-inflammatory properties. Pollutant removed is formaldehyde.

Garden mum

Inexpensive and widely available, garden mums love light and lots of water. They are simple to grow and care for, blooming through the fall months when other plants have often finished. Pollutants removed are ammonia, benzene, formaldehyde and xylene.

BODY: A checklist

Here is a summary of some of the things we discussed in this section entitled BODY.

Epigenetics:

☐ Epigenetics tells us we have more influence over biological expression and disease prevention.

Food heals:

☐ Reduce things that you know are bad for you.
☐ Eat things you know are good for you.
☐ Don't consume things that are bad for you - moderation is not an excuse.
☐ Make changes – ignorance is not an excuse.

Light therapy & Sleep:

☐ Use bright light in the morning from the sun (dawn simulator alarm clock or lighting box).
☐ Reduce blue spectrum lighting at night.
☐ Try the most unsexy glasses ever.

Supplements (with your doctor's permission):

☐ Adaptogens (teas or capsules)
☐ Omega 3
☐ Vitamin C
☐ Probiotics

- ☐ Magnesium
- ☐ Vitamin D (higher in winter, lower in summer, based on your test results)
- ☐ Vitamin A
- ☐ Vitamin K2
- ☐ GABA (if your doctor suggests you need it)

Exercise:

- ☐ Slow and easy walking that respects your level of energy
- ☐ Yoga
- ☐ Light stretching if yoga is too much
- ☐ Avoiding cardio (If you are burned out, give yourself permission to nurture the adrenals back to health.)

Health self-care:

- ☐ Get your Vitamin D level tested.
- ☐ See your doctor for a check-up.
- ☐ Reduce your toxic load.
- ☐ Get to know the "Clean Fifteen" and "Dirty Dozen" so you can choose foods that are less toxic.
- ☐ Check your hygiene products on the EWG database called Skin Deep and/or buy products that are less toxic.
- ☐ Add houseplants to clean the air at home and in the office.

Resources to check out:

- ☐ Dr. Terry Wahls: her TED Talk is life-changing
- ☐ Dr. Robert Lustig's YouTube lecture entitled "Sugar: the Bitter Truth"
- ☐ The "Food Babe" Vani Hari: lobbies the food industry to take toxins out of our food supply
- ☐ The Environmental Working Group: a passionate group of scientists who give us the straight goods on how to live in today's toxic world
- ☐ Dr. Alan Christianson's book, *The Adrenal Reset Diet*

Section 2: Mind

"Change your thoughts and you change the world."— Proponent of positive thinking,

Norman Vincent Peale

Epiphany (noun): A moment of sudden revelation or insight.

"An Epiphany is a visceral understanding of something you already know."— Success coach Jen Sincero

Ask yourself this question:

When was the last time I experienced an epiphany?

There is a reason that epiphanies often present themselves in the shower: it's because of mindfulness. In the shower, something incredible takes place: your awareness is drawn to your skin as you close your eyes while the warm water trickles over your face and down your back. In turning your awareness onto your relaxed body, an epiphany will often present itself. There is a lesson here: the solutions to our problems can often be found by removing our focus off the problem and onto BE-ing.

There is freedom in BE-ing.

I recall a time in my life when I would just sit and stare off into space, sometimes even cringing in boredom as I waited for a late doctor. Now I stare mindlessly at my phone and rarely feel a sense of boredom. I stare into my phone as if there is something of interest in there even though there isn't.

I can recall many times prior to having an iPhone, sitting at the doctor's office connecting with others, glancing playfully at children, smiling at their parents, giving up my seat for an elderly person and sometimes just dreaming about my life and solving the world's problems.

What does it mean to simply "be"? For me, it means accepting the moment for what it is without being driven to accomplish something, to be something, to create goals. It means to not be in a hurried state, and to remember what I am in all my greatness but including all my flaws. It means to stand tall as if I were a tree and uplift myself, and – hopefully without effort – to uplift others along the path.

In 2016, after I had been on Paleo for five years, I began to shift my focus from the health of my body to the health of my mind. Paleo had become my lifestyle, no longer requiring as much attention, and my body was functioning well.

I recently had an epiphany of my own.

I entered a room to join a person for whom I was providing personal counsel, and she said to me, "I feel better as soon as you enter the room; I am calmed by you." Like the impact of diet that I experienced by being Paleo, at that moment, through the practice of mindfulness and self-love, I experienced an incredible realization: I was making an impact on others around me; I could help others feel calm.

It felt good to have an impact on someone with such ease. For the first time, helping was becoming effortless.

I explored this deeply, really questioning my deepest desire to be a helper, and I realized that for many years I had attempted to help people who were stuck under a rock. But instead of helping them out from under the rock, I crawled under it with them. Sometimes I met anger with anger, and sadness with sadness. I felt their pain, and their pain was rubbing off onto my biology, presenting itself as burnout.

I grew to contemplate what true helping looked like, and reflected on what my true helpers were. This reflection brought me to awareness of three effortless helpers: a tree, a baby and a puppy.

What do these "helpers" have in common?

They never try to impress you, they don't try to help you, and they don't compare themselves to anything. They just are.

So ask yourself: Why or how can these things help? I believe the answer is about being connected or aligned.

As a life-long counsellor, parent, foster-parent, helper and friend, how was it that for the first time in my life, I was helping in a way that seemed effortless? I needed a deeper understanding of why; I recognized that I was helping effortlessly, but didn't understand what had changed. I had experienced such transformations that it was hard to know where, when and what had changed.

And then it hit me. This was my epiphany, my moment of sudden revelation.

It was self-love. In my centredness, I was in full alignment. I was resting in a place of self-love for the first time. I was in alignment with my truth, the truth of who I am and what I am, and the truth that my well-being is not attached to my successes.

One of the things we have probably all heard repeatedly is that you have to take care of yourself before you can take care of others. We know it's true yet most of us don't really do this. When we fly on a plane, we are reminded by the flight attendant to put on our oxygen mask first, because we would be no good to the toddler next to us if we passed out. We know we should eat more leafy greens, practice meditation more often or take time for self-care – but we don't.

Repeat after me:

My well-being is not attached to my success.

Command your body

Ask yourself this question:

Has helping been hurting my body?

Have you ever stopped to contemplate how you might respond biologically, physically, emotionally and spiritually to the various experiences in your life? Is it possible that your thoughts become your biology? I believe wholeheartedly that they can.

To truly transform the way we do things, and eventually improve them for the better, we first must undergo a certain level of self-reflection and self-awareness. Sure, most helpers tend to be self-aware on the emotional front. Most helping professionals learned about self-awareness in school, but this is something that needs to be ongoing. To focus not just on our emotional triggers and responses, we also need to zero in on the self-awareness of our physical and spiritual responses. When we encounter someone who's angry, sad or in pain, a person for whom we are providing counsel, how do we respond to their emotions? How do we respond to their pain?

Contemplate what thoughts go through your mind, what you feel, how this affects you spiritually and lastly, how your body responds to the experience.

I told my 15-year-old son, William, that I was writing a book and, as is typical for Will, he was rather unimpressed. I asked for his permission to discuss him here, in written form (which is, in truth, more about me than it is about him). He looked shy and embarrassed, and said, "No! What if my friends read it?" I told him that was highly doubtful since it's a self-help book geared towards helpers. As William walked away, he said, "It's fine, if you tell them I am 8 feet tall and VEERRY muscular!" So this is a story about my VEERRY muscular 8-foot-tall son …

William has been one of my greatest teachers. He has high-functioning autism. When he was younger, he had severe sleep issues. Growing up, he was on stimulant medications to try to alleviate some of the symptoms of severe impulsivity and hyperactivity. Despite trying to avoid medication for a long time, William could not function safely at school without medication. Each night, he followed a bedtime routine, which in all my experience and knowledge as a child-and-youth worker, told me was vital to bedtime success. I would have him soak in a soothing bath, sit quietly in a dimly lit room, read to him on his bed, and then without fail, things would go downhill. Even before entering William's room at night, I could feel my blood pressure rise, my heart race, and I would feel angry at the daunting task of putting him to sleep. I would enter the room, fully expecting a hostile exchange. Often, bedtime would trigger William to perseverate on the happenings of his day, stressors from school or life, like the time he cried for hours because we read *The Lorax* and he realized the injustice of all the "fishies" losing their homes. I can now look back on this with fondness and laughter, but at the time it was truly not fun. William would crash from coming off his stimulant medication, which would leave him feeling hungry, wired, hyper and – despite being tired – unable to sleep (a known side effect of the class of stimulant medication). I often had to give him food at 9 pm because another side effect is appetite suppression so he would often refuse to stop playing to eat enough dinner. Then at bedtime, once the medication had finally worn off, the hunger would hit. The exchange at bedtime was often an ugly scene of me being angry – not so much at him, but at the reality that at 9 o'clock when other 9-year old's were sleeping, I was there just trying to cope. I was overwhelmed by guilt and sadness, and in those moments things seemed hopeless and helpless. William's response to me had similar themes.

Many months after having gone Paleo, I completed a lab-testing hormone panel to see if I could delve into the next level of healing (ordered by my naturopath). In hindsight, the hormone panel revealed the not-so-shocking news that my cortisol levels were out of whack. It turned out they were elevated at night and extremely low in the morning.

Cortisol has been appropriately coined the "stress hormone," measured during several saliva tests throughout the day. A saliva test for cortisol is more revealing than a cortisol blood test which just indicates how much cortisol is in your blood at the time of the test. In my basic understanding of it, our cortisol should ideally spike in the morning to get us out of bed and pumped to face the day ahead), and slowly drop throughout the day to a very low level at night to encourage a restful sleep. People in the natural health community often call this the "cortisol slope."

My testing confirmed that I had a reverse slope, which meant I woke up every morning wanting to cry (because I felt utterly exhausted) while at night, I could barely sleep (because I was completely wired). It was as if my body had reversed itself and thought that night was morning and morning was night. The way I felt had everything to do with my lifestyle's effect on cortisol production.

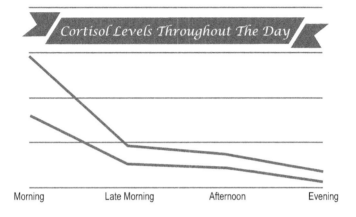

Cortisol Levels Throughout The Day

Morning   Late Morning   Afternoon   Evening

Despite all my attempts at a healthy lifestyle, stress was getting the better of me. Stress can kill people. I never contemplated the reality of my body being stressed – burned out even – I just felt that I was somehow above this reaction. I am almost always "cool," and I don't really allow things to get to me, except for my exchanges with my son. I always felt that my skill level in crisis management meant that I could out-play and out-wit burnout. Boy, was I wrong, and I had the test to prove it. My body was burning. This was a humbling revelation, to say the least.

When I heard this news about my cortisol slope, I knew I had to face the fact that, despite other contributing factors, the stress of putting my son to bed was a smoking gun. I knew I had to be less stressed about the task. I thought long and hard about my body. I longed to heal and I was on a path to having more energy and a less diseased-feeling body. I could feel a shift in realizing that the way I feel, the way I respond to my experiences, and how I think are all deeply related to my biology.

That night, I took deep breaths before entering William's room, deciding I was not going to get stressed. He looked at me almost expecting our nightly hostility but he saw that I was not agitated, and I refused to allow his mental state to agitate me. That night I commanded my body.

Boy, was it powerful. This was truly a pivotal moment in my healing.

William still felt stressed that night, but it was much less because I didn't add my own stress to the situation.

This was a light bulb moment: the realization that I could have autonomy over my own feelings and that as much as I love my son, I don't have to feel his pain or *be* his hostility. For the first time since my son's birth, I felt autonomous and I now allow him to carry his own burdens (while hopefully being a true support and guide to him).

My frustration in those moments prior to my autonomous light-bulb moment was about control. It was about resisting what the universe had handed me. I was living in the perception of injustice of what my son's path was. I was like a toddler on the ground kicking and screaming, wanting to control my life and the lives of those around me, falsely believing I could have more control than I actually had. I felt that if I worked hard enough, I could fix things for both of us. I felt angry at the knowledge that the obstacles he would have to overcome would be big and that sometimes even the smallest things would be hard for him. I wanted to control his behaviour, be the one to make him feel better and the mental health issue to just go away. I wanted to be the expert I had been for so many children leading up to that moment. I felt sorry for myself for having to watch my son in all that afflicted him and come up empty of solutions.

Lucky for me, wisdom is like rain – it fills up in the low places. These challenges led to the expansion of my wisdom.

I now know that surrendering, allowing and "BE-ing" is far more productive than grasping for control. I don't know why one child is born with autism and another isn't, or why some children have to fight cancer and some don't. I have lived long enough to know that life is not fair, never will be fair, and we shouldn't expect it to be.

Once I released the desire to control and for things to be fair, I felt free. I surrendered.

There is so much freedom in BE-ing.

When I entered William's room that night, I did help him. I supported him in his pain with a level of autonomy I had never known.

In this moment, I became the tree.

Repeat these words:

I can love another person and still have my own autonomy.

The following exercise is a strategy to command the body to remain solution-oriented. You will allow the other person to own their feelings, and you can eventually gain autonomy from them. You will command yourself to stay centred to who *you* are, not to what the other person is experiencing.

An exercise: Building awareness to command your body

1. Imagine you are sitting across from someone and they are sad, angry, overwhelmed or just generally stressed.
2. Take a deep breath.
3. Repeat these words silently to yourself: This problem exists outside of my body.
4. In this image, does your body respond to that person's emotional state?

   (You better believe it does. If that weren't true there wouldn't be such a thing as burnout.)
5. Think about your body in these moments; Is it stiff and tense?
6. Does your body "take on the problem?"
7. Command your body with the reminder that you are safe. Say these words in your head: I am safe.
8. Exert your control over your own body and your own breath.
9. Remember, this is not your anger, this is <insert person's name> anger.
10. Be aware of your internal dialogue in moments of crisis or even non-crisis.
11. Say these words in your head: This problem exists outside of my body; inside of me there are possible solutions or ways to improve this situation. It is okay for him/her to feel this way, and I will gently guide them towards possible solutions or improvements.
12. Keep your language autonomous.

Make some notes here about how this went:

_____

_____

_____

_____

_____

Did you notice anything? Resistance in the body? Resistance in the mind? Do you notice that when you focus on your breath it reminds you of the control you have?

As loving helpers, we sometimes think that absorbing the pain of another somehow helps them, but it doesn't. It's quite the opposite as we saw with the example of my years of failed attempts at helping William.

If you determine there isn't a solution, and often there won't be, just BE YOU, the person who resonates your true intention. In those moments, stop being a helper, someone frantically looking for solutions. And certainly, don't be someone trying so hard to be empathetic that you become a manifestation of their pain or fear. You may feel righteous to feel the pain of another, but stop doing that. Try to identify that moment in all your exchanges, that moment in your day, in your week when you became the manifestation of someone else's pain.

Think about it like this: People around you, particularly those you have been called to help, are trapped beneath a rock. It was not their choice to be trapped but it is sometimes their choice to remain trapped (or not). You are not required to crawl under to help them. If you do, you too will need help and before you know it, five people could be under that rock.

What that person needed was guidance on how to get out and validation of their trapped-ness. How on earth can you guide someone out from under a rock if you, too, are trapped?

To help someone, you must first help yourself.

Here's another truth …

> **Before you can love another, you must first love yourself.**

All of this, of course, is easier said than done. How do you prevent your body from responding when you see a person before you, deep in suffering?

One possible technique is to simply look for solutions. When you look at a problem, you tend to feel bad, because problems are stressful, but looking for solutions can be invigorating and fun. In your exchanges with others, try to highlight problems briefly, then talk with excitement about how to make improvements or even better, solutions. Don't get trapped in the vicious cycle of talking more about the problem than about the solution because that leaves everyone feeling despair, and helps no one.

Go back to the exercise earlier in this chapter …

Take a deep breath, remember who you are and remind yourself that "their problems exist outside of you." Tenderly, and with less judgment, look at them with concern. And listen. While listening, hear your own heartbeat and breath, and remind yourself to stay centred and that you are safe. Be the tree. Do this for you but also for them and the next person who needs you. Don't stress if you can't find a solution because not all problems have solutions. If this one doesn't have a solution, move your awareness onto something that does.

"You don't know what a big act is, it's not for you to know."

In other words, maybe you don't think you have the solution but maybe you solved something or inspired change that you won't bear witness to. Give up the control and stop trying to be superhuman.

Wounds of the helper

Let's talk about something that is rarely discussed.

In the helping field we often talk about trauma, acknowledging that childhood trauma has a profound and lasting effect on the brains of children, and exposure to this trauma leaves deep marks. Childhood trauma impacts key brain mechanisms, affecting mental health.

This is from the Child Welfare Information Gateway Issue Brief, April 2015 edition: "In recent years, there has been a surge of research into early brain development. Neuroimaging technologies, such as magnetic resonance imaging (MRI), provide increased insight about how the brain develops and how early experiences affect that development. One area that has been receiving increasing research attention involves the effects of abuse and neglect on the developing brain, especially during infancy and early childhood. Much of this research is providing biological explanations for what practitioners have long been describing in psychological, emotional, and behavioral terms. There is now scientific evidence of altered brain functioning because of early abuse and neglect. This emerging body of knowledge has many implications for the prevention and treatment of child abuse and neglect."

Most of us can acknowledge the lasting and profound effects that childhood trauma has on the growing brain; many of us have attended training seminars on this very thing. We learn about the pain and suffering of those we seek to help, of course, and we sit in deep thought over the pain of those we help.

To really delve into healing the mind and eventually healing the spirit, I believe there is merit in acknowledging the wounds themselves. If you cut your arm, it will require some investigation to determine the nature and depth of the wound and assess what it needs to heal. Maybe your wound requires stitches or needs pressure applied, or maybe it just needs some cream or a Band-Aid. Or perhaps mommy just needs to kiss it better (if you are 5).

Since we are all different when it comes to the state and depth of our wounds, this chapter will be kept short. But I do recommend pausing after this chapter to live in your wounds, acknowledging them so that in the coming chapters you will have a better understanding of what will help you and what might not.

Some wounds are by-products of professional therapeutic issues like transference, counter-transference and secondary traumatization.

A publication entitled "Substance Abuse Treatment for Persons with Child Abuse and Neglect Issues," provides a comprehensive discussion of therapeutic issues for counsellors: "Counselors also should try to keep a manageable caseload. They should deliberately set aside time to rest and relax, keep personal and professional time as separate as possible, take regular vacations, develop and use a support network, and work with a supervisor who can offer support and guidance. Some treatment settings have established in-house support groups for counselors who work with abuse and trauma survivors. By sharing graphic descriptions of clients' experiences with a colleague, the counselor can gain the crucial support and perspective to be able to continue effective treatment. Working as part of a treatment team can be a natural way to facilitate support and reduce stress."

This publication does a great job of identifying some of the issues that professional helpers face. The advice above is great in a perfect world, but fails to recognize that caseloads are rarely kept manageable.

In addition to being over-worked and facing therapeutic issues like those mentioned above, helpers carry a heavy load, they listen, love, cry, and often go into the depths of others' pain. They sometimes enter darkness that no person should have to step into: the darkness of the abuse of a child, of mental health, of our cultural propensity to sit back and do nothing about it. They bear this each day.

You have every right to be burned out. The job of a professional helper is one of isolation; confidentiality clauses make it challenging to really talk outside of work and when you do, you feel guilty. Most times you don't want to talk about the load you carry because you may prefer to numb the pain through distraction, food, denial, sometimes even substances. Slowly you may have transformed from a helper to one in need of help. It's important to talk about this, to identify the wounds you carry.

While suffering in the course of being a helper, many have also suffered in their own childhood. Being a helper can act as a deep reminder of these past experiences, which can add to the woundedness.

An exercise - Wounds of the helper

In this exercise, you will make a list of your wounds, of what makes your heart heavy. Take as long as you need but no more than a couple of days.

1. What are you angry at? _____

_____

_____

2. What makes you cry? _____

_____

_____

3. What makes you feel despair? _____

_____

_____

4. What makes you scared? _____

_____

_____

5. Write a list of your wounds, using one key word for each, separated by a comma. _____

_____

_____

6. Draw a stick figure

7. Identify, with a circle, where you believe these wounds are. (If you think the wound is so deep that it affects your whole body, circle the whole figure.)
8. Put this note aside for reference later in the book.

While it is important to validate and identify your wounds, don't spend too much time on them or you may inadvertently give them too much power. Acknowledge your wounds, but don't use them as excuses for not taking care of yourself. Don't use victim dialogue, or "woundology," if you will; it can become an excuse to not heal.

Ask yourself this question:

What will my world look like if I am healthy?

Rather than bonding over our wounds, we must learn to connect with one another over strengths. This goes for our connection with those whom we seek to help as well as the personal relationships in our lives. Be strong enough to be in the present, not the past or future.

Be the witness to the pain of others, acknowledging their difficulties with it, but don't spend too long in this state of witness in case you encourage them to be stuck there. Therapy, for example, is meant to be a ride from point A to point B, and point B should be a place of living past your wounds. Acknowledge the wound but recognize that the body, mind and spirit are meant to heal. You are not the person who was wounded, you are so much more now.

Self-talk & internal dialogue

"Our experiences, our stress, our food, even our thoughts eventually become our biology."
– Caroline Myss

An exercise: Self-talk #1

1) Give two examples of times you have failed or made mistakes. Preferably, they should be big to get the best out of this exercise.

   a) _____
   _____
   _____
   _____
   _____

   b) _____
   _____
   _____
   _____
   _____

2) Look past the mistake. Dig deep, past the pain of knowing you failed or that you could have done things differently and past the temptation to self-loathe. Live in the pain of the mistake, notice your ego's attempt to protect you by justifying your mistake or blaming another for their part in a situation. The ego will try to say, "so many others have done this too, I am not the only one." These are all ways that our ego shelters and protects us from the pain of knowing our mistakes – which can be a good thing. But it unfortunately stops us from delving deeper into ourselves, to tap into the wisdom that resides underneath our mistakes. It impedes the wonderful realization that our true well-being wasn't taken away by our mistakes, that we survived. More importantly we thrived and grew. Mistakes cause us to expand beyond who we were and transform us into who we are, which is a bigger, better, more enriched version of ourselves.

3) Delve deep past the mistake, smile in appreciation for your ego, your ruthless protector, as you sidestep it to find all the lessons attached to this mistake – the silver linings.

4) Record the silver linings with pride:

_____

_____

_____

_____

5) Compare these mistakes to a 1-year-old taking their first steps, and you will see how easily we: a) learn from our mistakes; b) become more skilled at being, walking

and knowing who we are because of our mistakes; and c) become balanced.

6) Now repeat after me: To these mistakes and all the mistakes I have made and will make, thank you!

Mistakes have been your greatest teacher. Love them and appreciate them. We all share in our experience of them; you are not alone in the mistakes you have made up until now or will make in the future. Mistakes are, in part, what you are made from. In accepting your mistakes, you will find it easier to accept the mistakes of those around you.

Say thank you to your mistakes. You walk because you fell. You write because you failed spelling tests in grade 3. You read because you repeatedly stumbled over words. You speak because you once babbled and made little sense. When you drive, you no longer speed (much) because of the time you (almost) got a massive ticket for speeding (that's me).

Now repeat after me:

To these mistakes and to all mistakes I have made, I forgive myself.

Along my journey to healing my mind, I delved deep into my thoughts, challenged my internal dialogue and shifted the way my mind was structured. I often felt as though I had little control over my thoughts and therefore my emotions. To some extent I felt as though I was a victim of my mind, like I was the passenger of some crazy bitch driving the car and all I could do was to close my eyes and pray I would reach my destination unscathed.

Albert Ellis, an American psychologist, developed a rational emotive behaviour therapy in 1955 which says:

> *"If human emotions largely result from thinking, then one may appreciably control one's feelings by controlling one's thoughts — or by changing the internalized sentences, or self-talk, with which one largely created the feeling in the first place."*

If language holds the power to deeply affect the experience of others, then language must also hold power over those who speak it. Your very own language defines your experience, not just the language that slips past your lips, but the language in your head. That language is the stories you tell yourself repeatedly, until you begin to feel the wrath of them, and the thoughts that you have been having over and over, until you seemingly have no control over them.

Vanessa Patrick, a professor of marketing at the University of Houston, discovered that people who merely replaced the words "I can't" with "I don't" fared better with behavioural changes. Saying "I can't" denotes a sense of limitation or constraint. Saying "I don't," on the other hand, asserts that you are in charge, and that is a powerful shift.

Try it for yourself and feel the difference.

I can't buy these shoes because I have no money.	I don't buy shoes until I have the money.
I can't eat sugar.	I don't eat sugar.

When you replace inner negative thoughts with encouragement you will be better able to overcome challenges. Small subtle changes always bring life changes. After all, keep doing what you are doing and you will get the same results. This subtle change allows you to feel less threatened and more inspired and interested in changing.

Chances are, if you feel a sense of disappointment, it's because your thoughts and expectations about a certain situation have set you up and let you down.

I have worked hard on this to find peace. I am a deep visionary who often lives in fantasy about how life will look, feel and be. To fulfil my fantasies of a certain situation, I often added expectation and pressure: for example, the many times I have fallen into Pinterest rabbit holes. In the past I would Pinterest "things to do for 14-year old's birthday," and envision myself as Martha Stewart. Without working up a sweat, I would easily transform my kitchen into something glorious. The cake would be homemade, there'd be balloons, birthday "cheer," and everything would match the colour theme.

After years of throwing parties for children, the most important thing I learned was that they didn't know or appreciate how much work, effort and money went into making those events happen. My efforts rarely, if ever, turned out like the vision. What made the party fun and successful was togetherness. My kids just wanted to be noticed on their birthday, and the vision was less about them than it was about me wanting to be a good mom. I was using those moments to confirm my place in their lives, to affirm my greatness, my love and my worth, especially as it pertained to my role as a mom.

Another one of my fantasies or expectations as a young mother was to sit by the fire on Christmas Eve and read to my lovely children "T 'was the Night Before Christmas." As I read to them, they would look up at me, all merry and bright, and we would be sipping eggnog. But that never happened even once. When I attempted to sit by the fire and read, they would fight, poke at me and say, "This book isn't fun, can we read another book?" I felt mad and upset thinking they didn't know *I* really wanted this. Quickly I changed my vision, nice as it was. We have seen this in the movies repeatedly: a twinkly, gorgeous vision of Christmas Eve which, of course, isn't real.

The media and the movies paint pictures that almost brainwash us into thinking that our marriages must be filled with lust from beginning to end, or it must signal an issue. We've been led to believe our birthday parties must be filled with shiny, plastic matching things to celebrate in togetherness, and we must go into debt to really celebrate holidays as a family. These are all lies, but there are more lies in your internal dialogue and your expectations if you look closely enough.

We all have expectations: what we want out of life and who we want to become. If you could reach a point where you were devoid of expectations, you would never be disappointed.

Having lower expectations about upcoming experiences allows us to accept the imperfections each situation inevitably has. Having fewer expectations of others allows us to embrace each person's imperfection. Having fewer expectations of ourselves allows us to embrace that we, too, are flawed.

Once I became willing to accept people for who they truly are and accept myself for who I truly am, once I became willing to accept the incoming experiences for what they truly were, I was handed a freedom like I have never known.

Acceptance is an amazing state of mind. When things do not work out the way we planned, it is so freeing to remember that this is how life works, rather than remaining in a place of frustration.

So if you want to avoid feeling disappointed, change your expectations.

A shift always begins with questions. Asking questions allows me to think differently and begs the mind to search for answers. A question begs you to look for solutions and reminds you that you are always learning with every passing day. How can you get answers to anything without first asking questions?

When you feel your peace of mind disturbed, ask these questions:

Why am I not at peace?

Can I look at this situation differently?

Can I look at this person differently?

Consider saying "you" instead of "I" because it is easier to ask yourself deep questions in the second person, and it beckons the helper in you to help yourself. It also provides a sense of autonomy and separation from the answers in a less threatening way.

This is the first step on the staircase leading you to your personal power. If you allow this, you'll be incredibly amazed at the shifts in perception that occur when you become willing to release expectation and see love and possibilities that reside in these shifts. When you focus on giving up the thoughts about how you imagined your life to be, you invite the most loving, truthful you to come forward.

Picture for a moment the idea of a child being raised without praise, never being told she is doing a good job, only being told she can do better. A child who is only corrected, yelled at and told he isn't good enough. It's a chilling thought; it's dark when you stop and picture it.

When was the last time you practiced self-praise? That too can be a chilling thought.

When we were in school learning to be various helpers, many of us were taught about "I messages," which help our remarks sound less demanding and blaming towards those with whom we are communicating. Of course, "I messages" have their place and do a pretty good job at helping identify feelings, but using them too much can fuel the ego and sometimes make us perseverate on our feelings and our entitlements.

Instead, using the words "we" and "us" will strengthen our teams, our relationships and our sense of belonging. They remind us that our feelings aren't the only important thing. Using those pronouns will remind us of our significant relationships and can increase our sense of belonging and purpose. They can remind us that we are needed as part of a system – small systems like families and large systems like organizations.

Language has the power to oppress entire minority groups. Words that speak negatively about the colour of skin, disability, religion, sexuality – words that are often used in jokes – can have powerful and lasting effects. They can be hurtful though sometimes not intentionally. But we recognize this power of language as being oppressive.

Why, then, do we deny this same degree of importance on our own slurs? "OMG, how could I be so stupid? This is going to take all day. I am never going to get this done! This is so hard, what if I don't finish on time?" Anger, sadness or frustration ensue.

Seemingly random, irrational over-reaction. We don't realize how negative thoughts can impact our mood, become obstacles in our path, and often lead to procrastination. Think of how many times you have put off chores you dread because they are going to take so long. You build up the idea of tackling the laundry to be more than it is, turning persistent thoughts into obstacles.

Our thoughts are closely connected with our emotions. What you think you can and cannot do is influenced more by you and your thoughts than the outside world.

An exercise: Self-talk #2

1. Write down five statements you say repeatedly that are not as positive as you know they can be:

   a. _____

   _____

   b. _____

   _____

   c. _____

   _____

   d. _____

   _____

   e. _____

   _____

2. Now rewrite those statements to more positive ones. Example: "I can't stand it when Judy speaks so negatively at work," to "Judy must be having a hard time."

   a. _____

   _____

   b. _____

   _____

   c. _____

   _____

   d. _____

   _____

   e. _____

   _____

Greatness

"Someone is sitting in the shade because someone planted a tree a long time ago."
— *American business magnate Warren Buffett*

Have you ever stood before a tree and been utterly moved by its greatness? Maybe you look at the tree and are reminded of God; you are soothed and touched by your creator. Or maybe you aren't a person of faith and believe in science; the tree touches you as you become aware of the beauty of our perfect symbiotic relationship with it. As the tree exhales, so to speak, you inhale. Nature put us together in this most perfect way.

A tree is selfish, never trying to impress you or compare itself to other trees. It doesn't care what you think. A tree is pure strength and love, and you feel that connection. A tree is greatness.

A forest is even more moving than a tree. We are that forest, a collection of utter greatness.

Now think about someone you struggle with, who perhaps "doesn't get it," or doesn't seem to be doing a good job. Maybe they just rub you the wrong way. What kinds of words are going through your mind? Perhaps it's thoughts about how they aren't good enough or their <u>lack</u> of greatness. Now take a deep breath and turn your awareness onto that person's greatness. If you can't, look harder. This person is as amazing as that tree that once moved you; you just need to turn your awareness onto it. Once you find it, hold on to it. If you haven't found it, keep looking.

This is about acknowledging the profound level of greatness that exists all around us. Imagine how wonderful it would be if you were able to turn your attention onto it. It has been my experience that by acknowledging greatness, you cause it to grow.

You are as great as that forest that gives us air and moves us all to be our best selves.

In David Suzuki's article for World Environment Day in 2017, he reminds us to reconnect with nature: "Studies show time outdoors can reduce stress and attention deficit disorder; boost immunity, energy levels and creativity; increase curiosity and problem-solving ability; improve physical fitness and coordination; and even reduce the likelihood of developing near-sightedness! ... In Japan, the term *shin-rin-yoku* — forest bathing or taking in forest air — describes the beneficial effects of connecting with the natural world. Japanese researchers have found people who breathe forest air lower their risk for diabetes and experience improved mood and lower stress hormone production compared to people exercising on indoor treadmills."

And there you have it. Proof that the tree really is an effortless helper.

Changing my lens through which I perceive the world around me to one of greatness has been one of my most incredible challenges and, without a doubt, one of the most rewarding.

If you look at the world expecting to find injustice, hostility, sadness, fear and pain, you will find it. Do you crave watching the news and staying current? Maybe that too is causing you to be in pain because it's all around us. Watching the news is tapping in to the collective pain of our world. How often have you watched the news where they covered the wonder, amazement and change that is happening in our world today?

If you look at the world expecting kindness, wonder, goodness, guidance, positivity, greatness, love, light, beauty and peace, you will find it.

Your perception and your awareness of your environment is all that matters. There is strength in all that saddens you, there is a lesson in all that angers you, there is greatness beyond the weakness you see, and there is love under the hate you feel. It is in the act of looking that it is found.

This practice – looking through the lens of greatness – beckons you to not only witness the revelation of your own greatness, but more importantly, to bear witness to the greatness of those who surround you. The strength, direction and wherewithal to only see greatness rarely just arrives at your door; you must go to it with the knowledge that it is there.

The most profound shift is sometimes done through the eyes, through the lens with which you see and interpret. Have you ever looked at a person and faked your approval? You look at them and act kind because maybe, on some level, it affirms you as a good person, or because it's the "right thing to do." But the deeper challenge is sometimes to dig deeper to reveal genuine approval.

The next time you speak to someone you don't approve of, consider reaching deeply, reminding yourself that it's not for you to judge and that sometimes the biggest act of generosity is giving another person your approval. As a helper, it is simple to support someone you believe in. The true challenge is supporting someone you don't believe in.

As helpers, we often find ourselves in scenarios where we are asked to support someone we don't believe in. How do you do that? Do you become an actor? In my experience, the only way to support someone you don't believe in is to find the belief.

Rise above anything that makes you not believe in them, acknowledge the times when you have failed to believe in yourself, and acknowledge your deepest desire for another to believe in you.

When you find it, you will emanate such a glow that that person will have no choice but to rise to the occasion, because you believe in them just as you have risen to the belief that you have in yourself.

If you need help carrying a heavy box, I can take one end to lighten the load and that's obviously helpful because maybe the load was too great for you to bear.

Through my years of heavy lifting at the gym, I would often look at my trainer and say, "I don't think I can," to which he would reply, "Jenn, you've got this." There is nothing like that feeling of accomplishment. He never helped me lift but showed me I could do it on my own, sometimes by walking me through the task, sometimes by saying "I believe in you." But often, just having him look at me through the lens of believing was enough to help me succeed and push to the next level.

We can lead someone in the right direction, like the proverbial "you can lead a horse to water but you can't make it drink." True helping is to be a guide, to show someone they can drink on their own, without you. I believe much of this guidance can be achieved merely though the eyes, if they reflect a tone that the helper is resonating in that moment.

Helping can be a slippery slope that can sometimes lead to the development of co-dependent relationships. Some helpers allow others to rely on them, to boost their own ego. I think it's better to lead through example, remind them it's their job to help themselves and give them tools, examples or exercises on how to do it. Look at them like you believe in them, or at the very least approve of them, because you do, because you've delved deep to find approval no matter what challenges they may be facing. Don't create a co-dependent situation, because true helping is walking them through their own uplifting.

Listening is what we do as helpers, but consider listening not with your ears, but with your heart. That's true listening.

Look through the lens of the eye with hope, possibility and belief; simply do not allow yourself a moment of helping without this intention.

Greatness is not an action, it's a place of being. Your actions are mere manifestations of the greatness that always exists inside of you and always will exist in you.

Whether you accomplish something or accomplish absolutely nothing from this moment on, you still have the power to move others.

You are perfect as you are. Be that, know that, and don't forget it.

An exercise: Greatness

1. Write down three things that are great about you:

    a. _____

    _____

    _____

    _____

    _____

    b. _____

    _____

    _____

    _____

    _____

    c. _____

    _____

    _____

    _____

    _____

> *"The purpose of life is not to fight against evil*
> *and misfortune; it is to unveil magnificence."*
> *– Inspirational author Alan Cohen*

Ok, let's chat. And please stick with me if it gets a little uncomfortable.

As I write this, it's 2018 and Donald Trump is in full swing in his time as President of the United States of America. On the day Trump was elected, I cried out of fear and anger. I cried not just because of my political leanings but because I feared that people really could be racist. I cried because I feared that LGBTQ people of America would feel and be unprotected, closeted, and hopeless.

On that election day I felt hopeless, sad and angry. I asked myself: "What if Donald Trump himself was cast to fulfil a character in the most grotesque play that I called *The Great Unveiling?*". True mindfulness in practice, which we will discuss later, is about calmly observing what is happening, knowing it will change. Change is inevitable, after all.

Act One, Scene One:

Could Trump be the universe's loving way of holding up a mirror to what we have become? Is that why we loathe him? Is it possible that he reveals to us the darkest parts of ourselves that we loathe? Perhaps the darkest parts of ourselves that we are in denial about? The darkest parts that deeply embarrass us?

Is it possible that Trump reveals to us the darkness, both individually and collectively, that we wish was not there? Unveiling our desire to segregate people who are different? Our deep racist ways that get swept under the rug, and all the many justifications that we create for this racism? The way in which both men and women perpetuate the deep trends of misogyny, as if they are woven into the very fabric of our beings? The way in which people use authority and money to derive a false sense of power and, at times, sexual pleasure? Our collective greed? Our worship of money that places it above all accountability? Our blatant denial of the state of our climate and our unwillingness to change? Our desire for power?

I asked myself some hard questions. I felt maybe this was like the moment in addiction recovery when they say "the first step to recovery is admitting you have a problem." Maybe this was our collective North American "rock bottom."

What can we do? How do we respond to this seemingly dark time?

We have chosen to make fun of Trump in the hopes of dissociating ourselves from him, and we put him down as if to say he doesn't stand for what I stand for. Perhaps collective self-reflection is in order and if you look closely, I think we are taking this opportunity to look at ourselves. I know I am certainly trying. I do not dignify this man's presence with my anger or fear, or by poking fun at him.

Through Trump and all people who challenge us, we are encouraged to ask these hard questions. We proclaim, as Oprah Winfrey does, "your time is up." Trump's presence in our lives, among other characters in the play of *The Great Unveiling,* has caused us to challenge many of these constructs that we have held on to far too long. These uncomfortable reflections are great catalysts for change. Great things have come out of this time, conversations are happening.

Let's allow him, and all uncomfortable people, to enter our path, to be the catalyst for change.

When Trump was first elected I was in a place of despair, resonating anger, loathing and, worst of all, fear. But I have allowed myself to see the good that exists in this experience, to reflect and eventually rise above any negativity that exists. Every time we poke fun at him, we participate and perpetuate negativity.

Act Two, Scene One:

Another character in our pretend play, *The Great Unveiling,* is artist Childish Bambino. This is the musical stage name for genius Donald Glover. In the spring of 2018 he released a musical masterpiece "This is America." It's a music video that is very political in nature, filled with artistic symbolism and hidden messages with deep meaning. It's painful, uncomfortable and certainly represents an unveiling. "This is America" holds up a mirror to display the grotesqueness that is America's reflection especially as it pertains to being black in that country. It asks hard questions and begs us to talk to each other, to no longer live in the belief that everything is okay.

Look around to see the cast of *The Great Unveiling* all around us.

This is the beginning of consciousness.

Our world is without a doubt in the midst of a great upheaval. We are begged to self-reflect because clearly, we have outgrown our current way of doing things. Change is almost always uncomfortable and sometimes downright painful.

In my 18-year career as a treatment foster parent, I stood before many children and youth who were filled with anger and rage. In those moments, the urge to meet those emotions with anger and fear myself was intense. But the best thing I could do was rise above that urge and look at them with the knowing that this was not who they were. Sometimes when we experience a raging and angry person, we have a tendency to respond with shaming them or making them feel humiliated. It feels natural to say, "look at what you have become" while shaking our head at them, but in most cases this doesn't help them, rather it makes us participants in the negativity. We cannot always see the best part of a person because often that part is deeply buried. I would say Donald Trump is a good example of this: when I look at him I have trouble seeing the loving being that I know exists inside of him. What if we all looked at Trump with that knowing?

The world may be broken, but this moment of brokenness is also beautiful. Existential crisis leads us to transformation, begs us – both individually and collectively – to reflect on how we can do things differently. This crisis will cause us to rebuild something wonderful, and now we can contribute to the dawn of that new age – the age of *consciousness.*

We can become alchemists and transform our experience of all people who we perceive as threatening, of the hate that permeates our culture, of all that is wrong, into a righteous one. Let's not give up, let's keep our eye on the ball of a new age of love and peace. Just like the aftermath of a vicious storm on the sea, the waters will calm, the sun will come out, the birds will sing, and we will rise again as a peaceful world.

But for now, this painful moment of change?

Repeat after me:

This painful moment doesn't own me. I own this moment. I will rise above.

What will you make of this moment?

Releasing fear

Ask yourself this question:

Am I motivated by fear?

There was a time in my life when I was living in fear. I was afraid of not always being a good person and I was tormented by what that meant. I wanted to be generous but I didn't want to be a pushover; I wanted to be kind but I didn't want others to walk all over me. The list of fears went on: I was afraid of being unsuccessful; I was afraid of messing up my kids; of being bad at mothering; of not fitting in but also of not being authentic to myself. I was afraid of other people's judgment; of being a slob or a bad housekeeper (in spite of being a neat freak); I was afraid of being unhealthy; of being fat; of chaos. I was afraid of spiders – okay, still working on that. But most importantly, fear had become the driving force in all that I did, in my every thought and action. And as I reflect, I realize I had always been driven by fear. This went beyond just chronic anxiety, this was a choice to live my life in certain boxes that I deemed acceptable requirements.

What a waste it is to live in fear.

Facing the fear involved rewriting my story, taking a big high-lighter and highlighting all that was right. It was about finding my breath, realizing that I have full control over my body and its reaction to my experiences. I can command my body, mind and spirit. Being "conscious," "aware," "centred" or "aligned" are the buzz words of our time, and for good reason because these things are first a choice but eventually become a place.

When I was resonating or vibrating the energy of fear in all that I did, I called more fear onto myself. The space around us and around our lives has a way of mirroring the very thing we put out. I was resonating fear, so fear is what I was bringing back to me, like a mirror. I had to stop directing my energy to the very thing I did not want. I looked out onto the world through the lens of insecurity and thus always being on the defensive against my fears.

Now, the things I try to call on with every ounce of my being, to resonate in every breath and every exchange, are love and respect. Respect for me, my children, my family, the people around me, and the environment. And what I find mirrored back in every encounter is true respect and love. It's wonderful. When I am a generous person, generosity comes back to me, every time. When I am a kind person, kindness comes back to me, every time.

When I first began to learn about the mirror I thought it was about action; if I "act" generous, then generosity comes back to me. This is partly true but I have learned that it's more about what I am genuinely feeling that is reciprocated. For example, if I perform a small act with real generosity in my heart, then real generosity comes back to me. On the other hand, if I perform a big act of generosity with a taste of resentment in my mouth, the results aren't as great. It's not about the action per se, it's about the energy you send out.

It's more about what is in your heart during an act than the act itself. We know this when we say it's the thought that counts. I would actually say it's the intention that counts.

Therefore, meditation is crucial to being aligned because we forget our genuine intentions, we forget who we are and what we are doing, and we allow fear to get hold of us. We must get back to BE-ing the tree, so that we resonate all the wonderful things we truly are.

There is freedom in BE-ing.

Psychological crutches can sometimes signal that we have buried fears. When a person sprains an ankle, the doctor often prescribes crutches to support the body on its way to healing and independence. An emotional crutch is similar.

In his article on the subject, Dr. Jeremy Sherman describes psychological crutches as "anything you rely on through vulnerability." He goes on to explain: "What you rely on could be chemical, emotional, intellectual, even physical, for example shopping or aerobic exercise when you're going through a psychologically painful breakup. And the vulnerability could be of any kind too, a breakup, a lost job, disappointed goals, aging, disease, even a sore hip."

Most of us use emotional crutches at some point or another. Even something as simple as crystals and essential oils that are geared to make us feel better emotionally can be crutches. Alcohol, drugs and food can also be crutches.

Sometimes we think crutches are bad so we want to rip them away, but if a person has a swollen ankle, would you do that? No, you would nurse the ankle back to strength.

What are your crutches?

What are you trying to mask?

Possibility

"Nothing is impossible, the word itself says "I'm possible." – actress Audrey Hepburn

Once I released my fears and crutches, what was left? Possibility emerged. Possibilities are endless: the possibility of living and being my authentic self, of becoming the most amazing helper who helps effortlessly.

Our beliefs become our possibilities. Think about it: any success you had in life began with you believing (at least partly) that it was possible. I didn't go to school to become a surgeon, probably because I didn't believe it was possible, but I accomplished many other things almost all of which began as a seed of possibility in my mind.

What you believe to be possible is what you end up with. Why would anyone enter a path towards anything if they didn't believe what they were doing was possible? Conversely, why would anyone take on a task they believed was impossible? When you talk yourself out of something, you're ruling out the possibilities with your negative beliefs before you can even try.

Ask yourself this question:

What is possible for me?

At this point in my journey, seeds of possibility were emerging but I still felt a sense of resistance to the new me.

My daughter Eden (William's twin sister) is 15, and she has given me permission to talk about her here.

Eden loves art, all forms of artistic expression, but specifically dancing. She isn't the best dancer who ever lived, but dance and artistic expression through movement has been her passion since she was 4 years old. Eden has always wanted to be a professional dancer but recently she feels she must be "realistic" about her future. She believes the life of a dancer is a difficult one, with shift work that seems inevitable in the industry, a lack of predictability and the uphill battle of generating an income. And she's uncomfortable with the grotesque way women's bodies are objectified in the dance industry.

Of course, these issues are all real. I asked Eden if she believed any dancers in the world have a steady income, if there are possible ways to generate income besides dance while keeping dance as a lifelong hobby and passion instead of only looking at our life's purpose as being income-based. I have encouraged her to look through the lens of possibility instead of fear, which looks at worst-case scenarios. Sometimes dreams are stolen from us before they can even take flight because we aren't looking at them in the right way. If Eden loves to dance, why does it have to be a career and job or nothing at all? Eden is learning from the outside world to follow her head and what is practical instead of following her heart and what is possible. I am not suggesting that she be unrealistic about her future employment and the need for steady income, but

I am suggesting we can follow our heart as well as our head in considering our future paths.

When I decided to write a book, I felt compelled to offer up wisdom and lessons as well as the story of my journey in the hopes it might inspire others. But I faced resistance, which looked a lot like Eden's "reality check" about what a dancer's life would be.

While this book is geared to helpers overcome burnout, I believe in the possibility that it will uplift someone outside of that audience. Instead of zeroing in on the impossible, I forced myself to focus on what *is* possible. The world is a mirror and if I stand in a place of impossibility, I will get the impossible every time. If, however, I stand in a place of possibility, the world will give me possibility.

Believe in possibilities. That's not to say you won't fail because failure is a part of life and is almost always a part of success. If you stop with every bump, then you are reinforcing your belief that it was impossible in the first place.

If you fall, keep going with your eye on what is possible, and keep reaffirming that you believe in your passion and yourself, by sticking with it.

> *"Don't fear failure so much that you refuse to try new things. The saddest summary of life contains three descriptions: could have, might have, and should have." – Unknown*

Your sac shall runneth over

You are filling a sac every day and you will have no idea until it's too late.

I want to tell you about a woman who had a deep, lasting and profound effect on my life. This is the story about a woman named Sherile (pronounced Cheryl), Sherile has my permission to discuss her here.

Sherile was a manager at my workplace, where her job was as tough as nails. resolving conflict and constantly putting out fires.

She was a passionate social worker, having committed her entire career to the foster system and the protection of children, which she tackled proudly, wearing her title like a badge of honour. I rarely worked directly with Sherile but as I got to know her, I was touched by what she brought to the office. Every time she was in a room, people vied for her attention. She was a dynamic woman with one of the biggest personalities you could ever meet; she was funny and bright, and so silly you peed your pants from laughter. She was a great listener and always made others feel like a part of a team. She also dropped more F-bombs than any woman I have ever met. Despite the challenges of her job, Sherile remained upbeat, continuing to laugh, joke, dance and sing.

But the impact of the stress over time was visible: Sherile was burning out and carrying brokenness.

Sherile had been part of the workplace for many years and when it came time to retire and say good-bye, she decided to move back to England to spend more time with her children and grandchildren.

I had the privilege of getting to know her a little over the course of about a year, but I was touched and amazed as her team members, co-workers and friends came together to celebrate Sherile's retirement. It begged me to reflect on what my life might look like at retirement.

As I saw Sherile wind down from her working life, I had a vision of a beautifully aged woman walking off into the sunset with a big sac slung over her shoulder, filled with "things." I was dying to ask what was in her sac, but I never did.

However, I think I know. I could see clues on her face, and from the absolute admiration and love on the faces of her co-workers, it was clear to me that she was leaving with profound and life-changing "things."

What *was* in Sherile's sac?

I believe her sac was filled with "light-bulb moments," with every time she made her co-workers laugh or smile, with friendships, and with wisdom too.

Inside that sac was the true knowledge of what really matters, the gentle sound of her friend Jen's voice and every glance of approval she got from her friend and boss Kathryn. It was filled with collaboration with her friend and office mate Cassi, and with every single connection, success and resolved conflict that she had tackled with integrity of her true purpose.

My guess is that Sherile did not take conflicts with her because she was so good at resolution. And that brokenness she carried – I think she left that behind.

I can see her walking into the sunset with her sac, wiggling her hips a little and humming these lyrics: "I am brave, I am bruised, I am who I'm meant to be, this is me." Bye Sherile, thank you for being my teacher.

Here are some of the lessons she taught me: Don't fill your sac with conflict. Don't fill it with bitching and complaining about some broken system or a boss who made you feel bad. Don't let each day be filled with anger or even the subtle annoyances that you might have trouble letting go.

Look hard each day at the things you want to put in your sac because in the end, you will care that you turned your attention to appreciation of all the enriching experiences life has handed you.

Every single moment of every single day, you are a student.

How did Sherile manage to change my life? I allowed her to. And now she is changing yours too, without you even meeting her.

You don't know what a big act is, it's not for you to know.

Sometimes you will see your impact, and sometimes you won't.

Every single experience is your teacher. Every friend and boss you ever have, your child, your co-worker and yes, even your enemies: those experiences are your teachers. Walk through life as a humble student, and you will leave with a sac filled with greatness.

Ask yourself this question:

What am I putting in my sac each day?

Venting is a good thing

Venting lets off steam.

I have this cool new kitchen gadget called an Instapot. I love this thing that does everything from sauté and slow cook to pressure cook, and has so many buttons I don't even know what half of them do.

My Instapot has a venting option and occasionally, as the pressure inside the pot builds, it releases a quick hissing sound. Without venting, my pot would surely explode. Just like that safety valve, venting can save us from exploding when our feelings build up.

Contemplate the difference between venting and complaining. For example, you could get something off your chest so you don't blow your lid or you could bottle up a negative thought about someone or something that keeps repeating like an old record.

How do we know when we are complaining versus venting?

When someone complains, they have consistent negative thoughts and small seeds of desire to change the situation but for the most part, they're unwilling to take action to set any change in motion. You know you're complaining because you're not really interested in feedback or suggestions, and you don't want to hear about the silver linings. Complaining tends to be repetitive and focused on the same thing. Complaining is draining.

Venting, on the other hand, feels cathartic. Much like the Instapot, it releases thoughts and feelings that we carry and need to articulate so that someone can be our sounding board. When we vent, it makes the problem at hand seem less daunting even though the venting itself won't immediately solve the problem.

I know when I am venting because afterwards, I feel lighter, I feel relief and I am uplifted. Most importantly, the person I have let steam off to isn't left feeling negative. In fact, they are uplifted because they can see that they have helped me feel lighter. That's why reliable friends and people are so important to our success as helpers.

Don't hide your negativity under the guise of venting. If you are one of those people who constantly engages in negative talk around the office, remember that it isn't helpful to you or your co-workers. Repeated negative thoughts will lead to burnout in a serious way for you and those around you. If you find yourself stuck in a rut of complaining instead of venting, here are some things you can do:

- Reduce your stress through yoga, meditation and deep breathing.
- Reframe your thoughts. Instead of having another negative thought about someone, think of three good things about her. What might she be struggling with? Tap into your compassion for her rather than disliking her.
- Distract yourself. Be compassionate with yourself and recognize that you are thinking negatively about a person because you are feeling overwhelmed. Take some time for you.

Ask yourself this question:

Am I truly venting or am I stuck in a negative space?

When I speak to people in my life about remaining positive in the face of adversity, there is always that one person who will challenge me and say, "Yeah but it's hard to stay positive when someone is an asshole." Yes, it is truly challenging.

I hold on to a deep belief that no one is truly an asshole deep down. Sure, someone can behave like it but I believe they are living only in the ego and have buried the best part of themselves. I try to look at them knowing that the best part of them is loving, even if I can't see it. Just like on the depressing cloudy days of November, when I can't feel the sun, I carry a deep knowing that the sun still shines.

I do this by being in tune with the best part, the loving part of myself, and being aware of how quickly and easily my own ego can turn into an ugly, raging lunatic. Road rage, for example, can bring out the worst in people. If I could make a bumper sticker it would be "let an asshole in," because even they deserve to be approached with love.

I knew I was onto something when it became easy for me to just allow an asshole to be in their negative resonance and to approach them with love. When you allow the assholes of the world to infect you, you aren't working toward the world peace or the inner peace that you want.

MIND: A checklist

- ☐ Epiphanies happen in the shower because I am relaxed and open to receiving.
- ☐ I can command my body, it just takes practice.
- ☐ I can love another person and still have my own autonomy.
- ☐ My worth is not in my accomplishment, it simply *is*. I am as worthy as a tree.
- ☐ There is freedom in BE-ing.
- ☐ I am wounded but I won't make my wounds the focus of my life.
- ☐ I will turn my thoughts into uplifting thoughts.
- ☐ I can, with practice, rewrite the script of my self-talk.
- ☐ I can, in time, help with less effort, the way these three helpers do (a tree, a baby, a puppy).
- ☐ I am great and I wear the lens of greatness in all that I do. This takes practice like exercising a muscle.
- ☐ I am releasing fear; it no longer owns me.
- ☐ Crutches are okay. I am in the process of strengthening my well-being and the crutches will disappear.
- ☐ Release fear to find freedom.
- ☐ There are endless possibilities in my life.
- ☐ What am I putting in my sac?
- ☐ I vent only when I really need to let off steam; I *think* before I vent.

Section 3: Spirit

We have walked through the body and mind; now we walk through the spirit which, for me, is leaving my mind for a time and entering my heart. To truly heal we must engage the heart.

What is spirituality?

Spirituality (noun): the quality of being concerned with the human spirit or soul as opposed to material or physical things.

What is spirituality? For me it means the belief that we are deeply connected. Call it nature, the universe, the source, a higher power or God: spirituality is about sensation, energy, vibration and resonance, all of which originate in the heart.

To command my body, I learned to engage my mind so that I could release the fears that had been holding me prisoner for so long. I needed my mind to rewrite my history and reassess my intentions. But getting to my destination was done through command of the spirit. I needed to activate my mind to get me here, and the practice of commanding the spirit is what keeps me here.

Existential crisis (noun): The moment at which an individual questions if their life has meaning, purpose or value.

Our planet is experiencing one of the greatest moments of upheaval; it is broken, seemingly shattering before our eyes. This is the greatest unveiling we have ever known – the unveiling of our deep cultural misogyny, of our global systemic white supremacy, the depths of our deeply woven racist ways, our greed, our desire for fame and power. Scrolling through news feeds has replaced reading real books; Instagram filters have replaced our canvas and brush; we don't value art in its natural beauty. We have lost eye contact and human connection. Our children are killing themselves and sometimes each other. Our collective systems are in pieces. The system of child welfare is broken, the system of health care is crumbling before us, our government is broken, our hearts are broken, our environment, economy, laws, children, spirits – all broken. We are in the grips of a collective existential crisis that we are a part of. We, too, are broken, and we contributed to the brokenness.

Is quitting an option? Of course it's not, because you care too much. The situation is dire and you are being called.

To fix our earth, our societies and our hearts, we don't need more security, police or military. We need real-time helpers and healers like you. This is our moment to save the planet, one broken heart at a time, starting with our own.

Existential crisis forces us to transform and begs us to reflect on how we can do things differently. This crisis is causing us to rebuild something wonderful, to reinvent ourselves and contribute to the dawn of that new age – the age of consciousness.

Is it possible that we are collectively stuck in a vicious cycle of trying to intellectualize our way out of our existential crisis?

Most people I talk to feel a deep knowing that things aren't right here on earth, in our country and in our hearts. We know that many of the systems that govern our lives are an ethical void, yet we circle around in our heads and minds, trying to intellectualize our way out.

Is it possible we are looking at it all wrong? Is it possible that we need to change what is in our collective heart?

We focus so much time on political correctness and trying to make everyone feel included but the root of exclusivity is not in our minds or policies, it's often in our hearts. Policy can change but until we address our broken hearts, nothing will truly change. *The Great Unveiling* illustrates this: we have been in our heads and intellectualizing many of our problems for decades, trying to make the world a better place, but it's not doing us any favours, is it? Look at the caricature of Donald Trump – what if he is the mirror reflecting our deep-seated issues back to us?

I believe that to heal this broken world, we need to get to a place where we love one another despite our differences. *The Great Unveiling* is happening, showing us the lies and a reflection that is so horrid we can barely stand to look. But we must face it, and instead of being defensive and closing our hearts to ourselves and the change we know is needed, we must open our hearts and love everyone as if they are truly our brothers and sisters. We need to surrender our need to always be right.

My personal definition of spirituality is to nurture the awareness of my connection to something bigger than me. My spiritual practice involves investigating the meaning, value, purpose and path of my life, and the acknowledgement that we are all deeply connected.

My interpretation of spirituality is not to be confused with religion. Religion can and should be a great thing, although I choose not to partake and hold no religious affiliation. The sense I have gotten from some religious structures is that followers believe there is only one path to divine connection

– a belief I think is held more in the ego than the heart. It can cause us to be separated from one another in a hierarchical sense, with a tendency for religious power to perpetuate the belief that its followers are somehow more worthy of salvation. It's an attitude that often excludes and insults other loving beings who walk the earth.

Energy, vibration, & resonance

We are not just bodies, we are also energy.

This concept allows us to act and respond from our heart and be guided by our feelings, our intuition and our inner knowing.

The heart is like a control centre. When we allow the focus of our awareness to be there, rather than being so concerned with the mind, there can be true transformation, and this is where freedom resides. This place is where YOU reside, the "all-knowing" ego-free you – the truth of who you really are.

You may think, what does energy have to do with anything?

Energy is everything.

Take a moment and think of a time when just being next to someone had an impact on you. Think about that time when merely being next to a tree had an impact on you. Being next to someone – like an innocent child playing quietly – can sometimes make you feel uplifted. Being next to an angry person, on the other hand, will often leave you feeling angry, especially when that anger is directed at you. Have you ever met someone and immediately knew you liked them, or found something calming about a particular person? The energy of the people around us can impact our own energy field, and we feel this every day.

Have you ever found yourself in a sketchy part of town where you felt scared or stressed even though there wasn't an actual threat presenting itself? We have all experienced these things and many other examples of energy.

We know energy well and can feel it often when we feel anger or love from another person. Love is not of the mind, it's of the heart, and it's an example of pure energy. How do you put into words the feeling you have when you hold a newborn baby? Or when you see a sunset that's so breathtaking, you take a photo only to look at the photo later and realize you can't feel what you felt watching the sunset. That's energy, which doesn't seem to translate in photo format.

What you are feeling is what you are resonating, what you are vibrating. Work on changing your vibration and you can literally change your life.

Life provides us with so many feelings: joy, love, gratitude, happiness – feelings so intense that they permeate your whole being. You can feel joy in every cell and molecule as you seemingly light up like a light bulb. In these instances, we explode with this incredible feeling which translates into energy.

The energy of our feelings is translated in frequency and vibration. Each feeling represents a change in frequency, like changing the station on your radio; one has loud heavy metal and one has gentle classical music. Each person holds a frequency. You acknowledge this when you say, "I had a gut feeling," or when you get a bad feeling about someone you pass on the street.

We have been made to believe that the mind is everything, that it controls us, but the mind is based in ego, whereas the heart is based in a deeper connection to who you are and what you need. Your heart always tells the truth but your mind can lie to you, like the times it has made you feel worthless. Your mind tends to make you feel like you aren't good enough, but your heart knows you are.

Try to become your observer by becoming aware of how you predominantly feel, assessing your thoughts and noticing where your attention is. Once you begin to control your thoughts, notice how you begin to feel more uplifted. **Become aware of your predominant feelings during experiences you are having.** Listen to your thoughts and notice how you feel when you think certain thoughts. Take note of **what happens when you direct your attention toward consciously feeling good.**

Stay present in the here and now, being aware of your thoughts and emotions, in your body and in your breath.

Paying more attention to your body, sensations and breath can create a powerful feeling of strength.

How can we increase our vibration?

It's easy to hold a high vibration when you're looking at the breathtaking sunset beyond the crashing waves with the warm sand beneath your feet while you're on vacation.

But how do we keep our vibration high when we aren't on vacation, in the midst of the hustle and bustle of life?

We've discussed many steps in the previous chapters: eating right, for example, improves your vibration because it makes your body healthier, while being in pain or having sugar addictions can harm our vibration. Everything in this book is geared towards increasing your vibration.

All things that uplift you are ways to increase your vibration. You know you are doing well because you feel better.

If you are depressed and become angry instead of depressed, you have increased your vibration. The goal with vibration isn't to be a happy-face emoji with rainbows and unicorns because no one is in a constant place of happiness. The point is not to hold in happiness but to hold the highest vibration that is available to us. If you have just lost your dog, for example, you aren't going to be happy. But you can live through the pain and work toward a better feeling. Imagine that our emotions are like a spectrum, with despair at the bottom followed by other feelings as you move up the scale, from anger and jealousy to boredom, hope and eventually joy.

There will be times when no matter how hard you try you cannot seem to improve your vibration, and that's where distraction helps. When you're unable to stop the circling in your head or get control over your feelings, try these tricks:

- Listen to an uplifting song
- Play a few rounds of Candy Crush, a repetitive game that takes some focus and can be soothing
- Take a hot bath
- Go for a walk in nature
- Get some exercise to get the endorphins working for you
- Start a gratitude journal

Here is a story about how family can evoke anger within us when we see them as reflections of things we once believed.

My friend was in a common-law relationship for over 20 years with a man who was a narcissist and rarely showed respect for her. Most of her friends and family knew she was deeply unhappy and devoid of a connection with her spouse. One day she mustered the courage to leave him, taking that hard step to become her authentic self and leave a place that didn't honour who she was. After the break-up, she settled into life as a single mother.

I felt proud of her although I knew single parenthood would be challenging. Eventually she began to date and put herself first for the first time in her adulthood. She eventually fell in love with a woman, which came as a big shock to her family. She called me, feeling stressed and seeking my counsel about how to face the fact that her family was not going to accept her new life. She was confused and hurt after finally becoming her authentic self only to meet resistance and anger from the people she loved most.

Here is my note to my friend on how to deal with others when they look at us as the previous versions of ourselves:

Perhaps your job is to surpass all that your mom has taught you.

Your mom's job was to provide you with a warm place to come into this world, and to pass on to you all that she knows, which may be in the form of what not to be. She is not required to come along on that ride with you, although she can.

Be sensitive to the fact that she may not have the energy to come with you in your growth. She, after all, went through the same long and exhausting journey, surpassing her own parents.

Allow her to be tired – at this point in her life she is not required to truck along as passionately as you.

Reaching a point of true emotional and spiritual authenticity is wonderful. It is exciting and enlightening, and I know that you so want your mother to come with you. You want her to leave her place of lies and shame and join you in authenticity and truth.

You lived in an unauthentic path for a long time because it was comfortable for you; it took such courage and strength to crawl out from there.

Maybe your mum doesn't have the emotional intelligence, strength or desire to join you in your new place. Be okay with her being tired; give her that permission. One day you will be tired and might not have the strength to join your children on their respective journeys, and you may have to say, "go on without me." And you will hope they will say with love, "it's okay, mum, I understand, I still love you for all that you have given me."

When you finally get to see the Grand Valley of Authenticity for the first time, stop and enjoy the view. Don't be sad or mad because your mom isn't seeing it with you because that will distract you from the incredible gift of what is right in front of you.

It's wonderful to have even small seeds of enlightenment (consciousness, awareness, awakening), to have obtained this level of authenticity; surely you could not have done this had it not been for those who raised you. A higher level of consciousness is something your parents may not yearn for, and that is okay.

When we believe in something that someone else doesn't believe in, it can evoke anger in us. Explore this for a moment by asking this question:

When you believe in something, why can it sometimes evoke anger when someone else disagrees with your belief?

I think there are a few answers to this question. We can feel afraid because if what I believe is untrue then I feel vulnerable. We can also feel angry because we want to control others to have the same perspective as us, especially when we truly believe we are right.

I have found this to be an amazing tool when anger presents itself over a differing perspective on politics or religion, for example. Just repeat this word: allow. Allow them to be who they are in their own path, and do this with the knowing that you truly want others to do the same for you. Allow me my thoughts and beliefs, knowing that my perspective is unique to me and you can't possibly know why I choose my perspectives or how they serve me. Don't tether yourself to others for the need to be right; in love, reach for emotional autonomy. When you feel angry at other people's perspectives, it's your ego, plain and simple. The real you would accept another's right to believe in whatever they want. In my experience anger is nearly always a manifestation of a fear.

When you are angry ask this question:

What am I so afraid of?

Then regardless of the answer, release and allow.

Somewhere along my convoluted path towards healing, I realized that I was listening to and partaking in agreements that no longer held truth and, in some cases, were based in lies.

Here are some constructs, some you may agree with and continue to partake in, some you may have already withdrawn participation in, some you may need awareness of:

Constructs you might tell yourself:

- I must be better.
- I am not good enough.
- I am not good, I am bad.
- I must deprive myself to be healthy.
- I need accomplishments to be worthy.
- My own greatness is to be feared.
- Money is my measurement.
- Intelligence is my measurement.
- Happiness is money.
- God is for the elite, not for me.

Constructs you might have allowed your parents to tell you:

- You are stubborn.
- You are weak.
- Expectations of what your life is or should be.
- Who you are or who you should be.
- You are smart but only to a point.

- You have always been someone who …

Constructs you might have allowed your church to tell you:

- You won't be saved.
- There is only one path to God.
- God is a punishing God.
- You are superior.
- You are inferior.

Constructs you might have allowed your neighbour to tell you:

- We are better because we have a nicer car.
- We are more successful because our grass is greener.

Constructs you might allow media/social media/society to tell you:

- You must be sexy.
- You are not sexy because there is only one way to be sexy.
- You must be skinny.
- Skinny is good but your breasts should be larger.
- If you are sexy you may be a slut, which is so unattractive.
- If you are not sexy enough you may be a prude, which is so unattractive.
- Sexiness is a measure of your worth but is unattainable for a person of your age.
- Girls are weak.

- Boys don't cry.
- Your body is an object.
- You don't have many "likes", therefore you are not liked; you must not be worthy of being liked.

Constructs you might have allowed the schools to tell you:

- Education is the only path to success.
- You can't get an education without us.
- We own your worth.
- Formal education inside the walls of a school is the only way to learn.
- Intellectual measure has the only bearing on your worth.
- You must be smart or you won't have a future.
- You would be broke without us; we are the only path to steady income.

Constructs you might have allowed your less supportive friends to tell you:

- You should be careful: that thing you are doing isn't the right path for you.
- You might fail.
- I am not sure you are cut out for this.
- I tried that and failed so you probably will too.

Constructs told by the government:

- A little bit of toxin is okay.
- Eat lots of grains or you won't be healthy.

- You need medication to prevent disease (like statin drugs).
- You are safe; we have a study to prove it.
- Those pesticides are harmless (we have a study to prove it).
- Cancer rates are rising because of meat consumption and individual lifestyle choice, not because of environmental toxins that we refuse to acknowledge.

The most crucial construct of all is reinforced through various systems:

- You are superior to anyone.
- You are inferior to anyone.

You already know that most of these are not based in truth, but do ask the questions:

How many of these do I invest in?

Do I participate in any of these agreements?

One of my recent challenges is believing at times that the universe is a punishing universe. Whenever a serious event happens, I find myself wondering if I am being punished. For example, when my son was diagnosed with autism I recall thinking, "I wonder if this is because I judged so many parents as a young adult that the universe somehow said, 'here's some perspective for you'." I don't actually believe, in theory, that this is a punishing universe but I do partake in this in practice, based on a keen awareness of my deepest feelings. This is about challenging who I am at the deepest core.

Think about the term "the apple doesn't fall too far from the tree." What does this mean? We have all seen this in action, which I think can be based on a constructed belief system. I have seen cycles of abuse and poverty, and children who have been sent to me from the "system." These children often come from generations of pain, trauma and suffering, from families who learned to live off the welfare system, believing there was no other way. I often tried to challenge these youth to see that there is another way of life. Every single youth who came to me from the welfare system was capable of being more but they partook in the belief that another way was not possible. All of us are stuck within our respective belief systems, which can stop us from being our absolute best selves. As a food coach, I saw morbidly obese clients who truly did not believe they could lose weight and then those who did lose weight still saw themselves as fat even after the fat was long gone. You are what you believe you are. You are what you believe you are capable of.

Challenge what constructs you agree to. As you walk through your life in the next few days, examples will pop into your consciousness and you will simply stop partaking in these things that you don't agree to, instead of walking around on autopilot and agreeing to things that contradict the truth of who and what you are. The truth of the world you desire, the truth of a peaceful world. Try not to feel angry as you begin to spot these lies and constructs that surround you. Be a passive observer at first. Consider which of these constructs are made up of truth and which ones are made up of lies. If you are confused, clarity is coming, I promise.

As I was on this path, I found that I ignorantly allowed this process to fuel anger in me. Don't fall for this. As you shift your awareness, your consciousness, to take notice of the falseness that surrounds us all, simply observe.

Let me clarify with an example: do you walk into your boss's office as their equal? Many of you do not even though you are their equal. So if you walk into your boss's office as someone inferior, this would be an example of a construct or a lie that you have agreed to, that is not based in truth. Because you are not inferior to anyone. A boss cannot make you smaller unless you agree to it. On the flip side, a boss can only be bigger if you agree to that too. Never agree to this; it's based on a lie. Your boss (a teacher perhaps) has authority over decisions regarding the organization that you are a part of, but your boss is not ever superior to you on a human level. If a boss tries to assert themselves above you, let them pound their chest, but do not shrink because the way you stand is within your control and no one else's. Don't meet this exchange of energies with anger or with fight. That is not what is needed to stand in your truth. Your boss is also filled with greatness but you are not elevating them to superiority if you notice them in their greatness. Noticing anyone in their greatness merely elevates you both.

Those things in your life that you are regretful about? Look hard enough and you'll see they are probably the root of lies you have told yourself, things you have done out of fear. The truth is, your past actions are not who you are or even who you were; you could say your expression at the time was out of alignment. The actions that you may regret, or that hold shame or fear, are not your truth.

Repeat after me:

Those things are lies; I am not that person.

Condemning yourself for past acts, belittling, berating or loathing yourself – these things reinforce the hold that lies and fear have over you. These things were done at a time when you were out of alignment; they are not who you are nor do they define you.

Fear claims more fear. Things that are done and held onto out of fear simply create more fear, and are manifestations of a lie. Dig deep enough into your fears and they are almost all manifestations of lies.

The good news is, the cages we find ourselves in are of our own creation. Lift your vibration beyond fear to align with truth.

One of the lies we have been told by the media is that there is only one kind of beauty. For women, this usually equates to skinny beyond reason, large perky breasts, small waistline, bleached blond hair, and a face masked by products. We are encouraged to buy products on every page of a magazine, every YouTube video advertisement, TV commercial and well-crafted store-front display. But this too is a lie perpetuated by our culture. The truth is, beauty need not be cosmetic. Of course there is beauty in transformation, inside the calm of our hearts, in nature; it exists all around us. We know that inner beauty is valid but do we really hold steady to this truth?

I love the word "awareness." Turn your awareness onto the non-cosmetic beauty that exists all around you.

Consciousness. Awakening. Mindfulness. Releasing the agreements that no longer serve you is a path to these things.

Find who you are and what you truly believe so you can know your truth. I promise though, this finding is not done within the mind, but within the heart.

Ask yourself this question:

Do I allow fear to rule my life?

I know the answer to that question is that you probably do live in fear because our culture, lives, relationships and structures all reflect how much we live in fear. You are fearful if you are clinging to the old versions of yourself, old agreements that no longer serve you.

Release them. You are not that person. You aren't even the same person you were yesterday. Once you know your truth, hold your head high, let your heart hum the tune that *is* you, and the fear will slip away. You will have nothing to fear ever again.

Sometimes the cages we find ourselves in are of our own creation.

With courage, leave the old and claim the new. Each day you are a new person, the life that you lived yesterday ends, and the new dawn begins.

Childhood influences and the people who raised us play a vital role in our upbringing. We must surpass what our experiences have taught us, take what we have learned from them, morph our interpretation into something better, and present that new expression to the world.

Face old, outdated agreements and reclaim your truth.

If we are going to reveal truth, we must face these lies for what they are, without fear, so that we grow from them, and release the structures we were led to believe. This process can sometimes cause anger and resentment. Sometimes there is pain, shame, embarrassment of the lies and sometimes we have a deep yearning for the past to have been different as we move through life with deep regret. Lies told about the roles we play, about the structure that life is, and the meaning that life must have. Lies about our potential.

Just to be clear: it isn't that lies need to be "taken down;" rather, the mere removal of our participation in them is enough to overturn most lies.

If you say, "Jenn is an arrogant, mean and selfish person," I can respond with, "But those are lies, how can they say that? Don't you know …" By responding in that way, I would become an accomplice to the lies just by entertaining them, I would dignify those lies with my energy and participation. Rebutting or debating makes me a participant. My best course of action is to rise above the lie and BE the truth.

An illustration of what I mean is this: How often have you seen a wonderful, uplifting article only to make the huge mistake of reading the comments section and being brought to your knees with anger, loathing, disgust or despair? It never ceases to amaze me how much anger we invest in internet trolls. Every time you feel anger, it's an investment. Every time you engage in a strange and pointless exchange with an internet troll you engage in a lie. We know they will not see your anger and change their stance. Yet they draw you in. Why? I know you don't think you can truly make a difference with this person hiding behind the comfort and anonymity of a keyboard. Ponder your vibration in those moments. Even if you don't respond to the internet troll and are just reading the comments, what are you "vibrating," what are you "resonating"? Likely, you are resonating anger at how they could be so incredibly insensitive to our world, and thinking they're an example of all that is wrong with the world. You use internet trolls to confirm your belief that the world is going to shit, that the world is a horrible place filled with pricks. But that would be a lie, wouldn't it? You know lots of nice people. So why are you allowing an internet troll to change your vibration? You give them a piece of you in those moments.

In any given moment, if you feel your vibration change from good to bad, repeat this statement:

I am allowing myself to feel this way.

Yes, you are in control and internet trolls can only spread fear and hate if we allow them to. Enter *Star Wars* music to remind us that we make a choice to be in the light vs dark. Internet trolls are basically the Darth Vaders of the world, but Yoda is everywhere – look for him.

The solution is simple: remove your participation in the lies. The hard part is that this includes your anger about the lies, your participation in carefully articulating and identifying them, discussing them, looking for them and wishing others weren't involved in them. Rise above to your truth.

Once we face the lies and claim our own truth, we find ourselves pulled back into the structure of lies that we have worked so hard to rise above, and this can cause anger and loathing.

Sometimes just being in our parents' presence, we unconsciously revert to the character we played as children and young people. When we are in the company of parents and siblings, it's almost expected that we play the same role we once did; if you don't play, you are shattering the lies for them in a seemingly alarming way, because they may not be ready to face the lies. They may prefer to live in lies where it feels familiar. When you change, it forces them to change, and they may not want or be able to.

If we refuse to play the expected role, they still see us for who we were and not our transformed selves. It can feel oppressive for them to only see you for who you were, which is a lie.

Sometimes we want to reject our parents, our family and the people who shaped us as children. We want to eschew any association with them because we fear that they reflect us, that we could become clouded by them. Sometimes we revert to the lies because they are so familiar, but we want to run the other way and never look back.

In transformation, we need to nurture compassion, stop blaming and simply proclaim truth: take back the truth of who we are as individuals and who we can become together in truth.

An exercise: Challenging your agreements

1. Refer to the list that you made in the exercise "Wounds of a helper."
2. Look carefully at it.
3. How many of your wounds were based on lies?
4. How many other lies have you inadvertently agreed to?
5. With each lie, state what the truth is. Example: I have always agreed to the lie that being skinny made me healthy but the truth is that listening to my body and eating food that makes me feel good makes me healthy.

Those lies are not you.

A beacon of truth

I love this time we are in; it is a time of universal unveiling – the unveiling of systemic racism, cultural misogyny, broken economic structures, and of the greatest environmental crisis of all time. So many uncomfortable things. We no longer have the privilege of sweeping them under the proverbial rug. Change is calling; if we want to be a part of the solution and the new age of consciousness, we have to become conscious of the uncomfortable truths. The truth of the part we play in the brokenness of the world.

As we reflect on everything that needs fixing around the globe, we see that the system of child welfare is no exception. Maybe you know this all too well after giving your life to child welfare and becoming one of the many burned-out victims of this precious life's work. Or maybe you've only just entered this environment and are filled with confusion. Perhaps you find yourself whispering in the corners of your workplace about bureaucracy and how senior management could do better. Even if you don't work in child welfare, your workplace is probably similar in that it needs help, especially if you are in the helping field.

I get it. You see that things aren't run the way they could be in a perfect world. Sometimes money is too vested in what we do or policy gets in the way of truly making a difference. We talk about "targets" and "professionalism," which detracts from the important work that needs to be done. We have heavy hearts when we realize our system is sending youth out on their own long before they are ready. The system, like most systems, is often filled with unfairness.

I get all of that. Many of these same things can be said for other systems within the helping field. Speak to nurses, teachers, first responders, frontline workers in outreach, community living structures, adult assisted living organizations: most workers in these environments feel we can do better.

What if, by holding on to the energy of the problems, you perpetuate them?

If you are walking through your workplace with an angry heart or angry words circling in your head (like, "what's the point?" or "sometimes I think we mess kids up more"), you are unwittingly a part of the problem. What if your fear and exhaustion breeds the very negativity you speak about? The purpose of fear and anger, after all, is to grow more fear and anger, like vicious weeds. The same could be said about positivity.

Let me take you back to the 1800s for a moment, with a passage on child welfare from *The Canadian Encyclopedia:* "In Upper and Lower Canada before Confederation, children were primarily the responsibility of the family. Any other assistance came from the church or from the local community. Provincial governments provided institutions like jails, reformatories and industrial schools, and support to orphanages run by churches and private organizations. They also established a system of indenture whereby a child could be assigned to an employer in exchange for room and board (and sometimes wages). At that time, most people in Canada lived on farms and family survival relied heavily on the work of children. When poverty and destitution, increased by industrialization and urbanization, took their toll, little public health or relief was available.

"Growing numbers of homeless, destitute children in urban centres, greater juvenile crime, and changes in child-labour practices pressured governments to respond to the plight of children. At the same time (1870-1925) large numbers of children were brought from Britain to Canada to serve as agricultural labourer and domestic servants. It was in effect the first large system of foster placement, and it often did not serve the best interests of the child. As philanthropic movements to rescue children from undesirable circumstances grew, organizations became larger and the state began to regulate and finance a system of child-welfare services. The first Children's Aid Society was established in Toronto in 1891, and the first Child Protection Act was passed in Ontario in 1893. This Act for the Prevention of Cruelty to and Better Protection of Children made the abuse of children an indictable offence for the first time. It also promoted foster care, gave children's aid societies guardianship power, and established the office of the superintendent of neglected children."

There is bureaucracy in all systems, often referred to as "bureaucratic bullshit," and for good reason, I suppose. In most helping fields, it can't be escaped and it will always be there. Our attention to it makes us part of the problem.

For a moment, consider what social workers in the above excerpt might have felt back in the 1890s, and acknowledge that you are here because of those who came before you. Without them this structure wouldn't even be in place.

You are part of a structure whose very DNA is the spawn of the people of our history – some very heroic people, I might add. They had far less, if not zero, paid vacation, probably very little sick time, and were forced to witness horrific conditions and standards for children in need of protection. Realizing a deep human need to protect children, they carried out a vision of a structure that would help those children. They heavily advocated for society to take notice that what was being done was not okay. If you are a social worker in child protection, that is why you are here, that is what you do and that is the essence of your life's work.

This ESSENCE is what I am getting at …

If you work on carrying the essence of your intention with you in all that you do, you live in the truth of what and who you are. When you live in the essence of bureaucracy you *become* that; you become the fear, lies and paranoia that can fester in those structures.

Work on drawing your attention to the uplifting changes that are occurring right now in child welfare. Recently the age of protection was increased from 16 to 18, something we have wanted in our hearts for years. And now we have it, the system is rising to continue to fulfil its original intention. Do you think that the people, the workers of the child welfare system had nothing to do with this change? Of course they did, they had everything to do with it. We all did. We spoke of our desire to protect older youth because we knew that 16-year-olds are entitled to safety too. Our beautiful system is listening and we must keep talking with an open heart.

Many of you are helpers outside of child welfare. If you work as a nurse, for example, you can go through this same exercise of looking to the past of what the structure of nursing was built from: healers – tender, kind people who helped others with pain and debilitating disease. Carry those original members of your organization's essence with you and, one by one, healing will begin to take place. As the saying goes, it starts with you.

This is consciousness.

Don't walk through the world unconscious and forgetful of your intentions. Don't close your eyes, smoke a cigarette, eat donuts, drink Coke, scroll through your news feed, make dinner and then go to bed only to repeat everything the next day. You are more than that, I guarantee. Perhaps you have just forgotten.

Resonate the original intention in everything you do. Making dinner? What is the intention? Nourishment. Remember your intention. Be the original intention of why you chose to be a helper in the first place. Be also the intention of the original building where you stand. Never has any social worker been in it just for the money or to make a broken system worse. Why then, did you come forth to be a helper? Be that. Remind yourself of that and it will grow, it will flourish, and others will catch on to your resonance. Doing this is incredibly healing; every cell in your body will thank you, each person you encounter will feel the consciousness emanating from you, and they too will begin to resonate the truth of their intention. When you live in truth, you give others permission to live in their truth. Don't allow yourself to perpetuate the lies that flow around you, don't even think about them or stress about them, just rise to live the truth.

As you stand in truth, becoming the essence of the true nature of what it is to be a helper, you become a beacon of truth and hope. You don't have to do anything but be your truth, live the essence, be the light, and you will lead others.

Perspective is everything

In May 2018, the auditory illusion on the internet of "Laurel versus Yanny" went viral. According to Wikipedia, after listening to the brief audio recording, 53% of more than 500,000 people said in a Twitter poll that they heard a man saying the word "Laurel," while 47% reported hearing "Yanny." The recording clearly illustrates how perception truly is reality.

If I look at my house where I raise my children and take such pride in ownership, I see it as my home. If you come along and for some reason see my home as a car, does your perception change my view of it? Does my home become a car? Of course not. But quite often the opinion of another does change our perspective. Take, for example, the shoes you love and think are nice: if someone says they're ugly, your view can change in an instant. So what is it: are the shoes nice or are they ugly? Perhaps they are both. At least not in fact but in perspective. Returning to the home vs car example, what if every person on earth decided to call a home a car: would I be angry? I might, because I know in truth that my home is a home and no one can tell me otherwise. But what happens to my anger, to my fight, if I "allowed" others their perspective of their truth – which may differ from mine – with the firm knowing that their perspective doesn't change mine unless I allow it to. And if they see my home as a car, is it truly hurting me? Only if I allow it to. Words don't change the essence of the truth of my home, which remains a home and something I stand in with pride. Your view of my home as a car holds zero power over my view unless I give you that power.

I am using this absurd example to illustrate that words can't change truth, but we allow them to by trying to exert power over other people's thoughts, opinions and perspectives. What I am really saying here is that the political climate right now fuels anger and division but only because we allow it to. We are being challenged to shatter our current belief system and structural agreements along many fronts including what gender means. One woman (Rachel Dolezal) even questions what it means to truly be black. Born and raised as a white woman, she now claims to identify as black. Many people remain angry with her because they feel that somehow, she stole something from them and that she hasn't "earned" the right to call herself a black person. These movements, these people begging us to question our reality and beliefs are awesome if we allow them to be, and if we don't approach them with anger. When something makes you question a truth, ask why it makes you angry. Ask questions, delve deep. Regardless of your political leanings, if someone asks you to partake in something you don't agree with, simply don't. Don't invest or participate in it, but please stop being angry with each other. If I meet Rachel, I will see a white woman and no amount of debate will change my perspective regardless of what she asserts as her truth. My eyes don't change her truth, our two perspectives can't touch each other and they don't hurt each other. But I would probably refer to Rachel as a black woman because she believes that this is who she is. I wouldn't meet her with anger because I haven't walked a day in her shoes. We don't have to fight about perspective. I can have mine and she can have hers. You actually can't fight about perspective because what you see is what you see and what you agree to is what you agree to. I agree to call Rachel a black woman but that will never change my perspective that she is white.

Just now I brought into your awareness some hot political topics by skirting past them. I am curious what you felt but more than that, I am curious how much you read the text in search of my stance on these issues. If you did search and I hadn't agreed with your stance, is there a possibility that you would have closed this book to disregard everything I've said up until this point? If you did search for my stance, why do you think you did? Are we searching to divide ourselves? If I had a differing perspective, might you have closed the book? I am challenging this because I have said many things you have may agree with, but when I bring up politics and possibly express a difference of opinion, this will often divide us. It will stop us from listening to one another. I don't want to argue politics here, but I do want to draw your awareness onto how much politics divides and discourages us from listening to one another.

If we want peace on earth, we must get ready to be uncomfortable.

The idea of simultaneously holding two opposing arguments in your head is referred to by psychologists as "cognitive dissonance." Psychologists suggest that doing this is so uncomfortable we will eventually choose sides. In the field of psychology, cognitive dissonance is defined as the mental discomfort (psychological stress) experienced by someone who simultaneously holds two or more contradictory beliefs, ideas or values. Cognitive dissonance occurs as a consequence of a person performing an action that contradicts their personal beliefs, ideals and values, and when they are confronted with new information that contradicts those beliefs, ideals and values.

It turns out we are wired to choose sides. No wonder we can't find peace. Maybe we must resist the urge to choose sides.

Do you believe that abortion is murder? If you believe in the right to choose, then likely you still believe that abortion at nine months of pregnancy is murder. So when does it become murder in this scenario?

No one wants to avoid these topics more than me, but I'm trying to illustrate the anger and the divide that politics causes. By embracing a little bit of cognitive dissonance, I have been able to tap into a deeper, more unconditional acceptance of people whose perspectives may differ from mine. It can be a great loving act. Yes, it can be uncomfortable, but fighting is something we have done often under the guise of "advocacy." What I am suggesting is that there is a third possibility in all our political divisions, and that is to try to live in another person's perspective and find some acceptance for it. Choose a topic on which you are firmly on one side of, and try to look at it from the opposing perspective even though that may be uncomfortable.

Maybe embracing cognitive dissonance is a brick in the path toward peace on earth.

Gratitude

"It is not happiness that makes us grateful, it's gratefulness that makes us happy." – Brother David Steindl-Rast, proponent of interfaith dialogue

Do you ever listen in on your thoughts and notice a trend?

In my interpretation of Eckhart Tolle's book, *The Power of Now,* he teaches about listening in on yourself without judgment, with the goal of separating from the ego. The concepts in Tolle's book are heavy, new-age stuff, but I highly recommend it.

The idea behind listening in on yourself without judgment has been truly miraculous for me. It has allowed me to really separate from my thoughts. Achieving autonomy over thoughts is an incredible feeling.

Separating from my thoughts has shown I am not my thoughts. And you are not your thoughts. Thoughts are powerful and important, yes, but for the most part we haven't truly exerted our control over them. We live under the false assumption that our thoughts just happen and that we have no control over them. But once we control our thoughts, we can eventually control our feelings.

When you hear your thoughts, and identify them as negative, stop and observe. Notice that when you become an observer of your thoughts, you begin to sense there are two of you. That other person is your ego. The ego isn't a bad thing; we all have one. We want to love our ego and acknowledge that it was meant to keep us safe. Our ego is the shallow part of us and we learn to live happily alongside it.

Don't be alarmed if, when you first listen in on your thoughts, you notice trends you didn't even know existed. (Like the time I realized I was overusing the word "infestation," usually in reference to rodents living in my back-yard deck, or harmless household spiders.)

The person observing your ego is the real you, the true you, the one without the need for all the social structures. That's the you that never needs to succeed a day to know your worth because, success is not something the real you needs to know, ever. That observer in you *is* the tallest mountain, the clearest diamond, the rarest gem that resides deep within you, me and all of us. That is where your truth resides. When someone held you as a newborn, this incredibleness was all that you were because you were free from ego. Even then, you helped because when someone holds a newborn baby they are helped by pureness, by the pure gift of love. This is the person I want to help you get to know.

The practice of gratitude is one way to begin to know the real person. As you observe your thoughts, try to reframe the negative ones into positive ones, by being compassionate instead of loathing yourself. Consider, for example, these statements that I have heard repeated in so many variations over the years: "How can I call myself a social worker?" or "When was the last time I helped anyone?" or "Aren't we just making things worse?" It is within our control to actively search for a better feeling-thought such as: "I enjoy going into the office each day and seeing Charles, he is so funny and such a friendly, loving person," or "I am so grateful to have a job, some people can't find a job."

This is about identifying truths that are more positive and feel better than the negative things that may also be true. We can all agree that there are things in our lives that could be better or, let's face it, that completely suck. This isn't about me trying to convince you that your life is butterflies and unicorns, this is about turning your awareness onto the things that don't suck and away from the things that do.

Sometimes the cages we find ourselves in are of our own creation.

Think about some of the relationships you have made along the way that perhaps balance out some of the negatives. There have been some meaningful connections, right? Every day, even when it seems there is little for which to be grateful, find something.

Gratitude is like a muscle; it needs exercise and attention. Practice gratitude in all that you do, and it will have profound and lasting effects on your life the moment you start.

Imagine you want to do push-ups, but you can't even do one so you start with assisted push-ups and work your way up to the real deal. Once you get better with practice, you will be experiencing real-life push-ups in the positivity department and your life will absolutely change for the better. Eventually you will be able to practise gratitude in all that you do, not just in moments of deep attempt.

When it comes to the pains of the past that you can't seem to let go of, consider changing your story, rewriting it word for word, thought for thought, until every negative thought is replaced with a positive one. There is always something for which to be grateful, something good that came out of the bad. Sometimes we want to resist or deny that we have the power to look on the bright side or find the silver lining because we feel angry, sad or let down by life. Challenges can act as stepping stones; they can hold us back or help us go on. Regardless of how challenging life gets, we always have the power to employ positive thinking. Always.

I have lived long enough to accept that life is not fair and never will be. Perhaps life was meant to be full of challenges. When we release the expectation of fairness, we feel less hurt, allowing ourselves to be in a place of optimism.

When in a helping situation and faced with a challenge, go back to the exercise in the chapter entitled "Command your body."

If you determine there isn't a solution, be okay with that. Try just BE-ing. Be a tree. The tree that you once stood before and felt moved by. Don't be a social worker (or whatever job title fits), don't be someone frantically looking for solutions and certainly not someone trying so hard to be empathetic that you become a manifestation of their pain. It may make you feel righteous to feel their pain, but stop, please. Try to identify that moment in all your exchanges, that moment several times in your day and week when you become the manifestation of someone else's pain. As helpers we do this.

There is freedom in BE-ing.

Let me walk you through what practicing gratefulness looked like in the beginning for me, so you can see how challenging this can be. As you read, see if you can spot two things: first, how I attempt to reframe every thought into a positive one (like exercising the muscle), and second, the two sides of me that always exist simultaneously (ego me and real me).

Deep breath …

I sit cross-legged with my back to the gas fireplace. My eyes are closed. I take a deep breath into my stomach. I am set to begin my gratefulness practice. I am excited and proud because I am showing up to practice what I believe in. I am relaxed, I am contemplating all the things for which I am grateful. Breathing! I am grateful for warmth, although my back is getting too hot. I adjust myself and move a little farther from the fireplace.

Why are my eyes open? I close my eyes again … Deep breath …

This practice is so great; it increases my vibration, helps me align and improves the overall contentment in life. It is almost spring, I am so grateful for the sun, for the yellow plum tree in my back yard, I can't wait for the white blossoms to come out. This gorgeous fruit tree is centred perfectly in my kitchen window, and acts as a backdrop while I cook in my spacious kitchen and wash dishes in my sink for the amazing family that I serve …

Oh yeah, I should throw on dinner when I am finished here … what am I going to make … shit, I forgot to thaw the chicken … okay, getting distracted …

I am so grateful for my privilege …oh wait, no, but I am not grateful for my white privilege … how can I be okay with that? Years of oppression that my race is responsible for inflicting ... I am not even technically white! Yes, but I live life as white so ... oh gosh ... getting off track ...

That tree blooms gorgeous white blossoms in the springtime which literally gives me goosebumps ... I am so grateful for that tree ... yes, too bad that one limb has fungus on it, oh man, we need to get out and prune that tree or the fungus is going to spread, why am I always procrastinating?

Deep breath, be grateful, Jenn, grateful.

I am grateful for the plums that the tree gives us every summer ... yeah, too bad the boys play basketball right near that tree and knock off nearly all the ...

Deep breath, back to centred ...

I am grateful for my children, watching them grow and learn, I just wish they would ... okay, stop, this isn't about goals, this is about gratefulness ...

I am grateful ... be grateful, you crazy ... you are not crazy, this is normal ...

For my hybrid vehicle, which is good on gas and good for the environment ... Oh man, I must clean the salt stains off the carpets – damn, that salt is so bad for the environment! OMG, global warming, the earth is dying, all the poor animals ... I wonder if I would survive a zombie apocalypse? Ha, who am I kidding? I would so not! Should we pack a bug-out bag?

Deep breath, be grateful ...

My vehicle, I am so grateful ... I need an oil change too, gosh there never seems to be enough time ... Winter tires ... is it too early?

Okay, let's start this gratefulness practice tomorrow, it seems I am not very good at this ... and I have *so* many things to do, oil change, thaw the chicken, Google yellow plum tree fungal infections.

No, you *are* good at this, you just must practice more ... I am trying to but ... you keep ... Ugh, DEEP breath.

Just stop thinking and listen to your breathing. Tree pose.

As you can see I need to exercise my gratitude muscle. This is comical, of course, but it's important to know that gratitude doesn't have to be done in this way either, it can also be done in smaller steps through-out your day.

I try to practice mindfulness and gratitude several times throughout my day, particularly in meetings when I am surrounded by smart people with whom I am collaborating. I love to collaborate with others and have allowed my heart to be filled with gratitude when I have the opportunity to chat with professionals and non-professionals alike. Particularly when I am in a room with other helpers. Writing this book has deepened my appreciation for helpers, and I love the moments when I am privileged to be surrounded by them. Today I met with a group of social workers – six women who have committed their professional lives to supporting foster homes. My heart was filled with joy and love when I sat back for a moment and consciously turned my awareness onto the fact that I was sitting in a room with people who, at the beginning of their adult lives, made a choice to become social workers. My awareness was keenly focused on what kind of women they must be to have set out to make a difference in their community. These are people who didn't choose money, they chose to make a difference. I told them what I was thinking and I am not sure if they thought I was crazy, but here is the point: never sit in a room with another and not contemplate the greatness that they are because if you do, you are missing out.

Change the story, the narrative in your head, rewrite it word for word, thought for thought, where every negative thought is replaced with a positive one. There *is* something to be grateful for.

Exercise: Gratitude

Make a list…

1. Feel-good moments _____
   _____
   _____

2. Good deeds _____
   _____
   _____

3. Acts of kindness _____
   _____
   _____

4. Things in your day that make you smile _____
   _____
   _____

5. Funny things _____
   _____
   _____

6. Beautiful things _____
   _____
   _____

I do this on my iPhone in the Notes app. I also like to write these things in texts to my friends, wife or children.

Forgiveness

"True forgiveness is when you can say, 'thank you for that experience'." – Media celebrity and philanthropist Oprah Winfrey

Rewriting your story and practising gratitude often requires forgiveness. Forgiveness is hard but it's essential to your alignment. After all, how can you be aligned to who you really are if your heart is heavy with anger and sadness? How do you release things from the past that have hurt you? You forgive for *you*, because holding onto this thing is not in your best interest. You forgive because you are worth it, because you know that you are in control of your feelings and no one else has that power unless you give it to them. Every time you do not choose forgiveness, you give that person or those people a small piece of you. By not forgiving you give them a piece of your future that belongs to you. You forgive because peace begins with you and if you deny forgiveness, you deny peace within you. If you want peace on earth, how will we ever get there if you can't forgive? It is within your purview to forgive.

Are you not forgiving because you need to know you were right? Don't hold on to pain because you feel like it somehow illustrates the rightness that you deserve. Only your ego needs to know you are right, the real you already knows the truth. The real you has zero doubt that a person did you wrong. One day, you may make a deep mistake and hope to be forgiven. Don't tether yourself to that person for the rest of your life. Have you ever been forgiven? Forgiveness is a gift you have been given by others many times. Life is a two-way street of forgiveness; it's all around you. People are constantly hurting one another for various reasons and offering forgiveness. Forgiveness is the gateway to your freedom.

> *"Forgiveness does not mean you have to accept the person back into your life or that you are condoning what they did. Forgiveness is giving up the hope that the past could have been any different." -- Oprah Winfrey*

Generosity

"No act of kindness, no matter how small, is ever wasted." – Greek storyteller Aesop

I found self-love in generosity.

The path to self-love was a path I didn't even know I was on. I believed I needed to be less generous, that I was somehow giving too much of myself, and that's how I became burned out. I began to exercise my right to saying "no." While I was nursing myself back to emotional heath, it felt good at first to say no. I tend to lack boundaries where helping people is concerned and I want to be generous to the point where I am exhausted.

Does this sound familiar?

The new self-care guru living inside of me started saying no. When a friend's father passed away, I thought I should make a casserole but that internal voice said, "you need to say no to this idea; you don't want to take on too much."

I felt bad at the idea that maybe we are all too broken to not be there for one another. I don't want to live in a world where generosity doesn't exist. Can we have both?

Eventually, I found balance to be the best compromise. I began to take on less, and developed a rule of "if I can help,

I will" and now, instead of making three casseroles, I make one. Instead of assuming I am the only one who can offer help (my ego), I encourage the person who needs help to ask other family and friends. Many small acts of generosity can help nurture a hurt person back to health.

I am a foodie who loves to feed people, but I realized that action and casseroles are not the only forms of generosity. You can give someone a fish, give them a fishing rod or teach them how to fish. Sometimes our words are a great gift of generosity. Sometimes, believing in someone with your eyes is just what they need. Sometimes, a person doesn't want you to solve the problem but just show them they are not alone.

Therefore, we can't possibly know what is a big act is. You don't always know how you have helped and in what ways you have been generous. Like the man who lived another day because of the woman driving along beside him, smiling and so full of grace: that moment changed him in the most profound way.

You do this too. Know it.

Being a generous person is truly one of the greatest sources of joy in my life and brings me a great deal of satisfaction.

True generosity goes beyond saying "let me know if there is anything I can do." To ask another person to humble themselves to ask for your help is falling short of true generosity.

When I see someone in my life dealing with stress or trauma, I will often give kind words, which is, in and of itself, an act of generosity. I will often say, "I wish there was something I could do to help," and sometimes I will give advice or listen. Sometimes I will try to merely meet the person's eyes with approval because that's what they need rather than help from an act of generosity. Be aware of what your eyes say to the people surrounding you; there is truth in your eyes and if you are giving someone a disapproving look, it can be hurtful.

Generosity to yourself is also important, so consider that perhaps the true act of generosity you can give some days is to ask for help for yourself. Putting aside your own physical, mental and emotional needs to be there for others helps no one.

I don't think I need to go into too much detail about being generous because chances are you have given so much of yourself. With the heart and spirit of a helper, you likely feel truly invigorated by acts of kindness and generosity, and you look for simple ways to do this outside of your helping field. Maybe it's giving a ride to someone without a vehicle or slipping a card with a thoughtful message into a co-worker's desk. The possibilities are endless. A small act will bring great joy and meaning to your life; it does not need to be a grand gesture.

> *"As you grow older, you will discover that you have two hands, one for helping yourself and the other for helping others." – Audrey Hepburn*

"Mindfulness is simply being aware of what is happening right now without wishing it were different; enjoying the pleasant without holding on when it changes (which it will); being with the unpleasant without fearing it will always be this way (which it won't)." – Mindfulness and meditation teacher James Baraz

Early in my path of self-discovery I held onto a bit of weirdness associated with new age themes such as mindfulness, consciousness and awakening. These themes evoked images of Buddhist monks living a life of celibacy and silence – people I didn't resonate with. Truthfully, I didn't even know if Buddhist monks were celibate or silent; that was a stereotype deep in my brain that wanted to hold me back from personal growth and awakening.

There were other deeply embedded stereotypes too: a highly flexible (usually skinny) vegan woman who did yoga and listened to chants while defusing organic tea tree oil and rubbing crystals to feel centred and connected. (For some reason she had moon tattoos too.) Clearly these stereotypes were not helping me; how could I buy into these new ideas with visions of people who didn't resonate with me?

Even the words "new age" caused me to raise an eyebrow in judgment of such practices. I had to face these false perceptions, wherever they were constructed in my brain or from external influences like the media.

We need to enter a New Age because things here on our planet in our collective spiritual avoidance simply cannot continue.

Following my transformation, I have happily become a stereotype as I stand in tree pose with a heart of gold, my eyes closed, meditating while defusing my favourite essential oil blend called "Cheer Up Buttercup,"wearing mala beads, yoga bracelets and "good karma charms," all with the knowledge that a New Age of mindfulness is approaching.

Our thoughts can be like a hamster running on a wheel, our mind trapped in a loop. This looping around and around causes us pain, anger, anxiety and resentment – you name it. Try as we might, we simply cannot stop the perpetuating loop.

Mindfulness commands the brain to stop and focus on what is in the now, whether it be the act of sitting, breathing, cooking or driving. Mindfulness allows us to focus on the present moment.

"To dwell in the here and now does not mean you never think about the past or plan responsibly for the future. The idea is simply not to allow yourself to get lost in regrets about the past or worries about the future. If you are firmly grounded in the present moment, the past can be an object of inquiry, the object

of your mindfulness and concentration. You can attain many insights by considering the past. But you are still grounded in the present moment." – Zen master Thich Nhat Hanh

Meditate, pray, be quiet with yourself and enjoy your own company. Listen to your thoughts, be aware of them and be okay with them. Be the onlooker to your thoughts, as if they aren't your own. This is life-changing. Don't *be* the voice but dissociate from it. You are not your thoughts, you are so much greater than those thoughts.

When it comes to problems, there's either a solution or there isn't, and if there isn't and you can't change it, then just accept what is. Sometimes when we put our problems aside, solutions come to us. New research has sent the U.S. Marines to explore how meditation can help people in the navy. Research is suggesting it can improve your heart too. Meditation has entered the scientific mainstream.

Neuroplasticity, also known as brain plasticity or neural plasticity, is the ability of the brain to change throughout an individual's life.

Our thoughts can change the structure of our brains. Let that sink in: your brain has the power to change. Crippling depression, anxiety that makes you feel frozen, irrational anger: these things can be controlled. Canadian researcher Dr. Lara Boyd held an amazing TED Talk on neuroplasticity, saying it takes 10,000 hours of practice to learn a new motor skill. So go easy, this is going to take time and practice. It's not just essential-oil-smelling-yoga moms from the suburbs who want to explore mindfulness. There have been some impressive studies like the one called "A Pilot Study of

Mindfulness-Based Cognitive Therapy for Bipolar Disorder," conducted by the University of Colorado.

Another one by Harvard Medical School in Boston on neuroimaging called "Mindfulness Practice Leads to Increases in Regional Brain Grey Matter Density" crushes the conventional wisdom that our brains stop growing and changing in response to experience. The study showed it's possible to reshape our grey matter in the way we do curls to reshape our quads and biceps.

It's no wonder mindfulness has become so popular. But what is it about mindfulness that changes us? I believe it is the fulfillment of a deeper spiritual connection that we all crave – a connection to the source within us. I'm referring to the deep indiscriminate, unconditional love that exists inside of you that was always there and always will be. The problems in our world are often managed by bombing, invading, bullying, buying out, etc. But the problems of our time cannot be dealt with like this; you cannot bomb the environment, you cannot invade a terrorist because you can't locate the target. Perhaps the universe is telling us something.

What is the lesson we must learn here? I am a big believer that problems present themselves to teach us. I believe the current lesson is one of love. We are spiritually void, we don't love one another, we compete with one another rather than spread love and kindness. If we loved our planet more, we wouldn't abuse it; if we spread love more, there would be a huge reduction in acts of terror. When a baby is denied love, that baby will fail to thrive. So will our planet, so will you and so will I. If we want to thrive, we need more love.

Sometimes we allow the problems of others to live inside of our body, which can lead to an ulcer, clenched jaw, sore muscles, rapid heartbeat or just plain stress.

Here is a mantra to bring you back to the fact that you are here to improve things, to think of possible solutions, but not to take on the problems of our world as your own. As you help, repeat these words throughout your day:

This problem is outside of my body. Inside of my body there is great love, great hope and wonderful possibilities, sometimes even solutions.

Various meditation techniques to consider

Breath Focus

Deep breathing, which promotes relaxation, is the idea behind breath focus work. It's actually as simple as it sounds.

Start by noticing your breath as you breathe normally. Then try a few deep breaths. The air coming in through the nose should be pulled into your belly. You can alternate between normal breathing and deep breathing. Truly observe in the moment and focus on your breath and the air as it comes in and out of the body.

You can also try placing your hand on your belly to feel the rise and fall as you breathe. Breathe in slowly. Pause and count to three. Breathe out. Pause for a count of three. Continue to breathe deeply in this sequence for one to three minutes, pausing for the count of three after each inhalation and exhalation.

Guided Meditation

Guided meditation, which is directed by someone else and is often practiced with relaxing music in the background, has become increasingly popular. Since guided meditations are directed by someone else, this is a great idea for people new to meditation. There are hundreds of guided meditations available on YouTube as well as many good ones on i-Tunes.

Deepak Chopra and Oprah Winfrey also have a "21-Day Meditation Experience" that's worth checking out.

If you prefer a more community-based experience to begin with, then look for yoga studios or wellness centres in your neighbourhood that offer group-guided meditations.

Visualization meditation

The mind is amazing and powerful and responds very well to imagery. In meditation, the mind concentrates which, in turn, relaxes the body. With visualization meditation, you engage the imagination to visualize images or ideas – kind of like fantasizing, in a way.

To perform a simple visualization, picture a setting, a person or sequence of events – something outside reality. You can visualize yourself there. One of my favourite meditations is to visualize myself on a beach – much cheaper than the real thing and no SPF needed!

Mantra-based meditation

The word "mantra" translates to "mind vehicle" or instrument. Participants repeat a word or phrase for the duration of the meditation, focusing on the mantra throughout.

During a mantra-based practice, when your attention drifts to other thoughts, you guide it back to repetition of the mantra.

There are many mantra-based meditations available online.

My favourite mantra, which originated with a French psychologist almost a century ago, is: "Every day, in every way, I'm getting better and better." You can also make up your own.

Loving-kindness or metta meditation

Loving-kindness meditation, also known as metta meditation, is designed to raise four elements of love: friendliness (metta), equanimity (upekkha), compassion (karuna), and pure joy (mudita).

The element of friendliness is expressed as genuine compassion sent out with the intention of surrounding ourselves and others with loving kindness. This can be sent to a respected person, a close loved one like a friend or family member, a neutral person and even a hostile person. With our yearning for peace in the world today, loving-kindness meditation is a worthwhile practice for each of us to spend time on every day.

When I practice loving-kindness meditation, I think silently to myself the following thoughts: "May I fill my heart with loving kindness. May I be at peace and at ease." Then I bring someone else into my awareness (a loved one and/or someone who I am feeling challenged by) and I will silently say: "May you be filled with loving kindness. May you be at peace and at ease." Then I bring all of humanity into my awareness and send the same intention out to all: "May we be filled with loving kindness. May we be at peace and at ease."

Forgiveness meditation

Forgiveness meditation is a way of opening yourself up to the possibilities of healing and love for yourself and for others. Its purpose is to release and let go of past actions that often have a hold on the present. This releasing and letting go can apply to resentment, anger or any number of negative emotions, so that your heart can heal and you can be at a place of true peace. Forgiveness meditation is a soft, gentle way of learning how to lovingly accept whatever arises and to leave it alone without trying to control it via thoughts.

In this practice, I settle in and take a few deep breaths, then visualize an image that represents a person I am in need of forgiving. I then label the feelings that come up as I think about this person: shame, anger, frustration. Then I gently call them by their name and bring awareness to my physical sensations, noting if I am tense or anxious. Keeping this person in mind, I will say, "I forgive you. I wish you joy and love." Then I take a deep breath and repeat this several times, breathing deeply between each statement. Lifting the burden of resentment and frustration from my heart is so freeing. Whenever I practice forgiveness meditation, I experience a lightness inside that is truly remarkable. This practice relinquishes the hold any person's action ever had over me.

An exercise: Mindfulness

1. Find a quiet space that is safe and comfortable.
2. Allow the landscape to be your backdrop, no matter how un-picturesque.
3. Close your eyes.
4. Concentrate your mind on the gentle noises around you.
5. Focus your attention on your breathing so that eventually it's all you hear.
6. Don't rush it.
7. Breathe in slowly through your mouth, all the way to the pit of your stomach.
8. Hold your breath for a count of 5.
9. Exhale slowly through your nose.
10. Repeat steps 2-8.
11. Imagine your breath is filled with an energy that is a healing life force.
12. As you hold your breath inside you, feel it renew you.
13. Release your breath and watch the toxicity of your thoughts and stress go out with your breath.
14. If your mind wanders, tell those thoughts to come back later.
15. Move the focus back to your breathing.
16. Do this for as long as you can or until your ass starts to tingle or the kids need yet another snack.

To truly grasp the exuberance of this moment, give up all attempts to possess it.

How many of these mindfulness strategies do you practice?

- ☐ Yoga
- ☐ Breathing exercises
- ☐ Cognitive reframing (positive thinking about what might help improve things for you)
- ☐ Healthy sleep patterns
- ☐ Meditation
- ☐ A hot bath
- ☐ Scheduling time for yourself
- ☐ Massage
- ☐ Exercise
- ☐ Prayer
- ☐ Being near a tree/forest bathing
- ☐ Holding a baby (if you can find one!)
- ☐ Positive friends (those who won't let you sit and bitch)
- ☐ Take control of a negative thought by distracting yourself from the problem with activities such as theatre, music, art, painting or crocheting.
- ☐ Positive self-talk and affirmations
- ☐ Remember that going from depression to anger *is* improvement.

☐ Have a sense of community.

☐ Do rather than talk: uplift someone by being with them (you don't have to talk to connect with others).

☐ Be connected – like the baby or tree that doesn't offer a word – and be an example of what true happiness is.

☐ Help and uplift others.

☐ A small act of generosity or kindness

☐ Do what makes you feel good. (Is there anything that makes you feel nice or good? Is there anything you can do to improve your feelings?)

☐ Practice praising and affirming statements: when you see a person reframe, distract or uplift, help them see it and praise themselves. Remind them that you would never consider raising a child without praising him or her so why not praise yourself.

☐ Praise yourself.

☐ Be an example.

☐ Wear a solutions lens rather than wearing a lens of problems.

☐ Make lists of pros in your life rather than comparing pros and cons. If you look at the cons, you radiate negative energy; only look at the positives.

Worth

> *"The energy of Gratitude is not 'thankfulness for something' but instead an awareness that every shred of life on this planet is a miracle, and therefore worthy of our admiration, our appreciation, our acknowledgment."*
> *– Spiritual counsellor and author Connie Kaplan*

When talking about worth, there is a tendency for the mind to go straight to "I know who I am" with descriptions like this:

- I am kind
- I am smart
- I am a mother
- I am a counsellor
- I do yoga
- I am a good friend
- I am funny

These things can be who you are, they can be your personality, but mostly they are your creations. They are constructs that you partake in to self-identify. WHO you are is your creation and it's an ongoing project, your masterpiece.

WHAT you are, on the other hand, is gold, magnificence. What you are is where your worth resides. What you are is all that matters. For a moment, consider what you are. It's a hard thing to articulate, so try to feel what you are.

What are you? You are not the façade that you've created but it may take years to answer this question. You will discover the deepest truth you have ever known about yourself and the best promise you have ever been told. I know the answer of what you are, of what I am, and I believe you do too, but you may have forgotten. You are a loving being. Regardless of what you have done, where you have been or what you think, you are a loving being.

To help you ponder that assertion, ask yourself to delve into the feelings you experience holding a newborn baby. Have you thought, "this baby is a bad person?" I am guessing you haven't. Usually the feeling you get holding a newborn is one of absolute, unconditional love. You hold that baby and you do not expect a thing from them. It's unconditional acceptance. But why do you fully accept a newborn yet hold so many conditions over everyone else, including yourself? My experience of holding a baby reinforces how quickly I can be in love. It reinforces the notion that I *am* love, and that every single pore of my being can spill with love and acceptance for another, especially when I erase the illusions of "conditions." With the newborn, you become the giver of love and in that giving, you receive, like a mirror.

Every one of us was at one time a newborn baby. That thing that evokes unconditional love in most of us – we are still THAT.

One of the practices that encourages me to engage my heart (and get out of my mind) is to place my hand on my chest. It reminds me to feel my heart, to lead with my heart in all that I do. My mind doesn't control my actions, it is almost all based in ego, but my heart, on the other hand, has never let me down. If we want peace, we must start with peace in our hearts. Let the heart guide you.

Back to worth ... Repeat these words:

My worth is not in the helping of others. My worth is not my accomplishments.

Your accomplishments are not your worth, it's not in how much money you have, how much organic coconut oil you eat, the diet you follow or the number of squats you can do. You simply will not find worth in an outside space.

You are worthy because you *are*. It's that simple and yet that profound. A baby, a tree and a puppy never look for their worth, but they are certainly worthy. They never try to help you, and yet they do so without effort. If we want to be the best helpers we can be, we need to learn from these three great helpers.

I have heard miraculous stories (granted, on some strange YouTube rabbit-hole viewing session) about people who've experienced near death. I have heard them say they are changed, and all their problems seem trite compared to the miracle of life.

Stop for a moment and think about some of the incredible things the universe provides us: water, mountains, sunsets, birds, warm breezes, beaches ... life on earth *is* a miracle.

You might not see it if you are wrapped up in the past. Sometimes we worry about how we didn't do this or didn't do that, we focus on our failures and the failures of others, and we reminisce about the fun we once had.

You might not see life's miracle either, if you focus too much on the future, thinking about what will make you happy or what you wish for. The present is all there is and all there ever will be. Consider stopping to smell the roses in the present. Presence is the greatest gift you can give yourself and another person.

An exercise: Holding in your worth

1. Picture these things:
   a) Uplifting birdsongs in the spring
   b) Playfulness of kittens
   c) Stunning rainbow-coloured fields of tulips
   d) Rushing waters filled with life
   e) Powerful bolts of lighting
   f) Breathtaking mountain landscapes
   g) Golden sunsets
   h) Warm southwesterly winds
   i) Alluring canyons
   j) Giddiness of puppies
   k) Lush gardens
   l) Twinkle of the stars
   m) Powerful claps of thunder
   n) Crisp autumn air
   o) Hot and hazy summer sun
   p) Rage-filled storms
   q) Glistening of the northern lights
   r) Wonderful orchestra of the forest
   s) Stunning untouched glaciers
   t) Fury-filled rushing river water
   u) Preciousness of a newborn baby
   v) Untouchable Milky Way
   w) Crunchy autumn leaves

    x) Blazing full moons

    y) Bright shining morning sun

    z) Richness of soils

2. *Really* picture them.

3. Go back and read the list again if you need to.

These things all bring me to my latest life lesson: the most intense spiritual lesson thus far and the one I am just beginning to wrap my head around.

It is the miraculous and stark revelation that when I deny ME, when I deny that I have purpose and deny my worth, I deny the whole universe, every single thing on that list. Think about that.

The life force that created you, the love that *is* that force, whatever vital cosmic reasons are behind your creation – that is your purpose and your worth.

When you contemplate the vastness that is that force and the power behind that decision, there must be unwavering belief in your purpose. There must be such a knowing of your purpose. When you deny or refuse to believe in your deep, meaningful purpose and the deep meaning that is you, you deny the intelligence, force, strength, power, love and omniscience of the entire universe itself. You deny all the things that gave you a sense of connectedness in the above list along with everything else in the universe.

Let's take this a step further.

If denying your self-worth and purpose is to perversely deny the whole universe, then surely denying that any other human being holds purpose and worth is also to deny the whole universe.

Every single human being holds purpose and worth, otherwise the omniscient power would not have created them.

My truth as I experience it doesn't have to be your truth. My spiritual path doesn't have to look like yours. We were created to reflect diversity so the path to the truths we seek will also be diverse.

Higher purpose

> *"A hero is someone who has given his or her life to something bigger than oneself."*
> *–Scholar Joseph Campbell*

I want to walk you through my own spiritual transformation that occurred over the past several years.

My life is pretty ordinary; I am not extraordinary or special. I have discovered some truths. Along my path, there is one main theme I want to share.

I have been looking for love, for worth, for many things, but I never found any of those things *outside* of me. To find love, I must BE love, to find worth, I must BE worthy.

You ARE love, you ARE worthy, these are your unwavering truths.

Authenticity is a trendy word right now. What does it mean to live your authentic truth? Is your authenticity in the clothes you wear? In your closet? In your accomplishment? We know it isn't but we don't always live it.

You are your authentic self, you are truth. You will not find authenticity outside of you; it is inside.

When I think of prayer or spirituality, I sometimes feel closeted, because I am embarrassed that anyone would assume I am religious or that I think I am superior in some way, that because I have a relationship with the universe I will be saved but you won't. I find this so ridiculous. So the thought of coming out to my readers as someone who prays admittedly embarrasses me a little. Religion can often be used as a structure of the ego that seeks to make one person or group of people more powerful over another. Since I grew up non-religious, most religious traditions seem strange to me. But somehow, having a relationship with the universe never seemed strange to me in the slightest.

I spent much of my childhood begging for breath. I grew up with severe asthma and frequently had attacks that sent me to the ER. The household I grew up in had smokers, we had a cat and a dog, and my asthma was completely out of control for most of my upbringing. I always felt unattractive because I was constantly blowing my nose, had permanent dark circles under my eyes and shakiness from the medication. My breath was almost always bad from the constant inhaler use. I can remember often feeling as though I might not take another breath, that this one may very well be my last. In every one of those moments, I prayed. I never fell to my knees or bowed my head, I just closed my eyes and asked for help. I listened for strength and direction and amazingly, strength and direction came every time.

My whole life, I took for granted the sense that I truly was never alone, but that a strong cosmic force was there for me at every fork in the road, every stressor, every crisis.

When I entered my adulthood, having this strong cosmic connection helped me follow my heart and find love in partnership and the greatest love I have known in my children.

I always had a deep sense of direction to go where I was being led. My life always seemed right even at the lowest points.

I was shocked and confused when I realized as a young adult that some people didn't feel my life as a lesbian was a righteous life. That somehow the love I had found was not real. I even had someone (whom I love) suggest that the love I feel is the "devil in disguise." No wonder I felt closeted about my divine connection; to align with that shit was deeply disturbing to me. I was getting messages like, "your love is the devil but my love is from God," and "God is love but only mine, not yours," and "my marriage is meaningful and yours is meaningless." How could people think this when this powerful force was beside me my entire life and giving me deep approval the whole time? While I would be lying if I told you these realities have not been painful, I remind myself that perspective is everything. I try as hard as I can to face the discomfort of my own cognitive dissonance and look at it from others' perspective. I believe that the perspective of those who seek to make my love less meaningful is based in fear. Holding on to that truth softens my heart and allows me to experience love for my naysayers instead of pain or confusion or, perhaps most importantly, anger and fight.

Returning to the subject of my severe asthma, when I was 22, I had an attack after having the flu, and one of my lungs collapsed – very painful. I had an x-ray to rule out pneumonia and after looking at my results, the ER doctor gasped in horror. He said, "I don't think these are yours! These look like the lungs of an 80-year-old!" I recall him double-checking the name and my hospital chart and bracelet. He couldn't believe the amount of scar tissue on my lungs.

I am happy to report that in January 2018, for the first time in my life I was breathing on my own without the use of steroidal inhalers. I believe I am healing on a cellular level through food, exercise, the power of managing my thoughts and maintaining positivity, through my spiritual practice, and by maintaining a deep knowledge of WHAT I am.

The disease called asthma – that thing in my life that seemed at times like the worst thing, that I can be mad at or sad about or that I could have felt sorry for myself about – may have been the very thing that brought me to the deepest connection I know.

Suffering isn't always what it appears to be. Your enemy can be your teacher, your suffering can be your healer, the one who has brought you the most sadness can be an angel in disguise. Open your heart and mind to other possibilities.

I will end this chapter here because I am not sure that I am ready or willing to delve deeply into my relationship with this strong cosmic force in such a public way. I have trouble speaking about this without religion getting in the way, without divide getting in the way. I still have so much fear to release in this area, obviously. I also think that the path to this deep connection is profoundly personal and differs from person to person. And I want to respect that many readers may not be interested in this discussion. I am hopeful that if you are someone who yearns to develop or deepen your relationship with a higher purpose, you can open your heart and begin with listening and asking.

Self-love

> *"What lies behind you and what lies in front of you, pales in comparison to what lies inside of you." -- Ralph Waldo Emerson, essayist, philosopher and poet*

As I walked you through my path, you can see that this journey has been one of deep self-discovery, amazing transformation, epiphanies and great life lessons. At every step I delved to deeper places within myself. I challenged my body to be better, I challenged my mind to think differently, I challenged myself to be a better mother, wife, person and ultimately, helper. The truth of what I was looking for all along was, however, none of these things.

Self-love is the true pot of gold at the end of the proverbial rainbow. We have been trying to justify or intellectualize deeply to land in a place of self-love. For me the destination of self-love hasn't been about delving into or working through issues that began in childhood; ironically, true self-love began when I stopped trying to work through anything, trying to use intellect to find my worth, justifying who I was, making goals about how to be a better person, or analyzing the self that I had become to sculpt it into a better version of me. True self-love came in the instant that I stopped all self-discovery. The landing of self-love has been in the quietness of the mind, in the breath and in the act of simplified being. It's in the knowing of what I am and why I am, it's in the compassionate lens of seeing my imperfect and vulnerable self with an open heart, and it's in the cessation of correction.

It's hard to walk another person through my journey to self-love because it hasn't been a linear path. But what is self-love anyway? How do you obtain it?

Self-love is not to be confused with self-care. Self-care is part of self-love but it's not the full picture. Self-love is a loving place to be, especially if you have spent many years caring for others and neglecting yourself. Self-love is, and should be, a priority. To truly help another human being, you must first be aligned with your true self. The more you focus on your well-being, cultivating and nurturing it, the more confidently you will be able to stand before someone with a problem and experience their true upliftment.

On the journey to self-love, resistance will creep in, especially as it pertains to what other people think. Do not resist landing in a place of self-love because you're afraid of what people will think. What they think does not matter; it only matters if you say it does.

Repeat after me:

It does not matter what people think about me.

Sometimes, I draw pictures in my head about what people might think of me. I wonder what they think about how I look, what I say, what kind of mother I am, how smart or even how dumb I am. I sometimes assume that others judge me or don't wish me well in all that I do. I think that some people don't believe I'm worthy of being "saved" because I don't partake in their religious constructs.

All of this is resistance that no one but me put there. Every obstacle along this path was me.

Let's face it, every person in my life and everyone who knows me may or may not have thoughts about me. I am the only one who has to walk in my shoes, and every moment I spend thinking for other people, being paranoid about what they think of me, is a waste. The only one I ever have to think for is me. At some point, I decided to assume that everyone would accept me for who I am.

Don't assume you know what other people are thinking; let them think for themselves.

This book was the first step on that course. Imagine writing down all your deepest beliefs and walking through your journey in book form. Nothing has made me feel more vulnerable than that.

I can't tell you how many times I envisioned various friends reading this, and thinking, "oh no, I wonder how she will judge me," or creating perceptions about what others might think of me. I know I shouldn't care and that when I envision what others are thinking, I am turning myself over to fear and participating in lies rather than holding steady in my place of truth. I know the truth: that I am not responsible for how others feel, only for how I feel.

When I hold steady to my truth, I walk into a room with my head held high without analyzing the landscape in search of approving eyes. I no longer live in the lie that I need another to rescue me. I stand firm in the dis-owning of others' feelings. I reach for true autonomy and release the need to make myself small in order to make others feel better. I release the need to change my tone or my words to avoid offending. I ditch the egg shells under my feet for a stance that is unapologetic and firm in who I am, accepting myself as a flawed being, accepting my ego and my journey, all with a loving spirit.

Whenever I feel resistance creeping in, because it will, I remind myself to *be a tree*. With that reminder I know that I don't have to do or accomplish one single thing; my worth is in standing tall, it's in my breath, heartbeat, smile, laughter, eyes and in the lens through which I, and only I, can see.

If you are unsure of what action to take, ask yourself this question:

What makes my heart sing?

Self-love is not a constant state. It is small moments in each day, in moments of reflection on the years passed, and the overcoming of heartache. It's in the getting up after a fall, it's in generosity, forgiveness (of yourself and others) and accomplishment after having faced resistance. Self-love is in the pursuit of your dreams, past the voice that told you you couldn't. It's in perseverance. Self-love can be found in a long list of natural wonders and small pleasures: babbling brooks at the bottom of a mountain; the deep breath after a long hard day; a baby's small foot; a puppy's excitement; the wind in the trees; the moon and stars; fresh glistening snow; the creativity that flows through you to your keyboard; your paintbrush as it strokes the canvas; the realization that you are unique. It is in chocolate cake, passion, warm breezes, birth, death, new and old. It's in who you are, who you were, and who you will be.

Just look.

Repeat after me:

I am the only thing standing in the way of my birthright to REST in a place of self-love.

> *"Love is the great miracle cure. Loving ourselves works miracles in our lives."— Motivational writer Louise Hay*

Practice makes perfect

Now that I have walked you through my journey of transformation, I hope you will consider taking some baby steps toward your own transformation. The key to change is in changing your practice. Consistency is mastery.

> *"I fear not the man who has practiced 10,000 kicks once, but I fear the man who has practiced one kick 10,000 times." – martial artist and actor Bruce Lee*

What is your practice? What has your practice become?

Mastery follows consistency. You can master being the best helper you can be by consistently showing up for you, by nurturing yourself like it's your job. Everything you do *is* your practice. What you choose to look at, from Facebook and Instagram, to Netflix and the evening news, is your practice. Everything you listen to – music, talk radio, the lady down the street – that is your practice. Everything you think, the circling in your head about the annoying guy sitting next to you on the train – yes, this, too, becomes your practice. It's all your practice in thought and in choice. What you put on your skin is a practice. Even the way you breathe is your practice.

What is your practice?

What do you eat? What do you think? What is your focus? What do you desire? Do you desire? Do you even allow yourself to desire?

If everything you think becomes a practice, and everything you eat becomes your practice, then when you change your practice, you change everything. Change your practice and you will transform.

Align your practice with what you value, with what you want. Align your practice with who you truly are, not the person you constructed in lies and ego, not the person you constructed for your own "safety," not the social you but the real you. The real you is not the one you made smaller because you didn't want to offend or the one that is so buried in other people's desires or wishes or the you that is lost. When you make yourself a priority, you make everyone around you a priority. When you find peace within yourself, you contribute to the dream of peace on earth. BE the change you want to see.

To practice moving through the world in a conscious state, you must:

Pause. Breathe. Remember who you are. Remember your intention.

Tomorrow when you forget and become unconscious again because life got busy or an asshole crossed your path, repeat.

Pause. Breathe. Remember who you are. Remember your intention.

It will be a bumpy road and you will fall along the way. The key to all that I have done successfully up until this moment was in not giving up.

> *"We have hardship without becoming hard. We have heartbreak without being broken."*
> *– South African human rights activist Desmond Tutu*

It's not that life in my newly transformed practice is perfection, it's that I can finally experience heartbreak without being broken, hardship without becoming hard.

Oreo cookies. You like them. They are crispy on the outside and soft on the inside. You like the taste but when you eat them you feel guilty because you likely believe they aren't good for you. You may have falsely convinced yourself that everything is okay in moderation (and you know how I feel about that lie!) and say you're just going to have two. But before you know it you've eaten a whole row. I think it's safe to say this act does not align with what you believe. You do not believe that Oreo cookies are good for you.

Every single moment of every single day is a choice: a choice of what to eat, what to do, where to go; what to notice, ignore or think; what to feel, plan or believe; a choice of who you are and what you stand for. To be the you that you want – the you that you desire – you must align your practice with what you believe to be true.

Align your actions and thoughts with your beliefs; when you become firm about this, you transform yourself.

Through my entire life as a helper, I felt the need to convince others to believe in their worth and in healthy eating. Now I think differently; I believe that everyone is already filled with desire and belief but they have not aligned their practice with those two things.

It is not me who needs to convince you. *You* need to align the who-you-are, *you* need to show up for you and not just for others. You may falsely believe that your actions are aligned with your beliefs under the guise of doing for others. By now you know this is the lie we have lived as helpers and it serves no one.

Helping others by being selfish and loving yourself allows you to become the greatest example. You stand strong as a healthy, vibrant, loving, rooted tree, and *that* helps people, *that* is peace on earth.

We have walked a small journey here together. I believe with all my heart that the steps in this book are a small contribution to peace. Peace begins within, with me, with you. Peace lives inside of us all.

We have talked about burnout in the context of helping, we have talked about other great helpers – the tree, the baby and the puppy. We have talked about the healing powers of food, what we put into our bodies, what we see, what we breathe. We've covered light therapy and supplements, mindfulness, venting, commanding our body, seeing greatness all around us, and being a beacon of truth. It's not enough to simply learn about all the things you can do to heal your body, mind and spirit. It's not enough to simply believe in these ideas or steps. I know likely you believe in most of this.

The convincing is, in fact, the easy part. Just like eating your vegetables, you don't actually need to be convinced of these principles to know these steps will likely be helpful to you.

Now you must show up to practice what you believe in. If you believe in mindfulness, then why aren't you showing up for the practice of mindfulness or meditation? If you believe in eating your vegetables, why aren't you eating them? If you believe that you are what you eat and what you think, then why aren't you changing your food and your thoughts? All you must do to see change is to simply change the practice of what you are doing.

Ask yourself this question:

What baby step will I take today toward peace?

SPIRIT: A checklist

- ☐ My spiritual practice is mine, no one else's.
- ☐ There are agreements that I partake in that don't align with my truth; it will take practice to identify them.
- ☐ Once I identify an agreement that doesn't align with me, I merely withdraw my participation.
- ☐ I can be a beacon of truth.
- ☐ My perspective is mine; no one can change it unless I allow them to.
- ☐ I do not need to feel angry if others have a different perspective. Allow.
- ☐ I am gratefulness.
- ☐ I can forgive and it's the most loving thing to do for me.
- ☐ I am mindfulness.
- ☐ I stand in the knowledge of what I am (a loving being).
- ☐ I am on the journey to my higher purpose (and perhaps always will be).
- ☐ I am generous.
- ☐ To love myself first is the most loving thing to do in an act toward peace.
- ☐ Every day I will take baby steps toward the practice of the person I want to be.
- ☐ I am consciousness.
- ☐ It does not matter what people think about me, it matters what I think of me.
- ☐ What makes my heart sing?
- ☐ I am the only thing standing in the way of my birthright to rest in a place of self-love.

Epilogue

Releasing this book is like releasing my diary for all to read, partly because I feel that my spiritual practice is private, it's deeply personal and doesn't require sharing with others. I never saw that deep cosmic force as needing praise outside of my deepest genuine gratitude and servitude. What I choose to resonate is my praise. What I choose in action is my servitude. This experience didn't require articulation until I felt it did, until I felt my experience may be an inspiration to others. Releasing these words for all to read is by far the most vulnerable thing I have ever done.

As much as I love myself, I admit I still hear voices – perhaps now mere whispers – of doubt, that people will judge my path or my truth. These doubts act as proof that my work here is incomplete and perhaps always will be.

My truth doesn't have to be your truth.

This is a note to you, the reader and helper: in my heart, as I wrote these words, you were this person:

When I first met you, you represented hundreds of others who had come across my path before. Like I once was, you were broken. You were aging, I could see the lines around your eyes, the dehydration of your skin, your tired gait. Despite being so visibly burned out, amazingly, your light still shone through so brightly; others could see it, I could see it. You never ceased to make others laugh, you never stopped responding to the people around you who were still asking for your help in various ways. As I sat with you, your phone would buzz with activity, you always read the messages with genuine concern, and often stayed late at your job to respond to those in need. You were tired and your body inflamed but you were still so beautiful and kind, and I am so grateful to have met you. Please take the time to put yourself at the top of your list of priorities, if not for yourself, then for the many people who will need you in the coming years. If we are deeply connected, and I believe we are, then to help another is to help yourself; as another succeeds, so do you.

As you begin your transformation with small changes over time in all areas of your well-being, you begin to take on the role of director in your stage experience, you begin to realize that you have power in the well-choreographed dance of your body, mind and spirit and the miraculous expressions and manifestations that will, no doubt, come out of that.

Now go eat some vegetables, would you?!

The End.

References

Preface

"Burnout." Merriam-Webster. Accessed May 26, 2018. https://www.merriam-webster.com/dictionary/burnout

Brown, Brené. April 30, 2018. "Courage Over Comfort: Rumbling with Shame, Accountability, and Failure at Work." Brené Brown blog. Accessed May 26, 2018. https://brene-brown.com/blog/2018/03/13/courage-comfort-rumbling-shame-accountability-failure-work/

The helper

"Help." (verb). Oxford Advanced Learner's Dictionary. Accessed May 26, 2018. https://www.oxfordlearnersdictionaries.com/definition/english/help_1

Ronald Reagan quote. BrainyQuote. Accessed May 26, 2018. https://www.brainyquote.com/quotes/ronald_reagan_120491

Section 1: BODY - Header page

Jim Rohn quote. PassItOn.com. Accessed May 26, 2018. https://www.passiton.com/inspirational-quotes/7279-take-care-of-your-body-its-the-only-place-you

Epigenetics

"Epigenetics." English Oxford Living Dictionaries. Accessed May 26, 2018. https://en.oxforddictionaries.com/definition/epigenetics

Bell, Chris. "Epigenetics: How to Alter Your Genes." Oct.16, 2013. The Telegraph. Accessed May 26, 2018. https://www.telegraph.co.uk/news/science/10369861/Epigenetics-How-to-alter-your-genes.html

Food heals

"Dr. Terry Wahls: How to Beat Progressive MS Using Paleo Principles and Functional Medicine." April 4, 2017. Ancestral Health Radio. Accessed May 2018. http://ancestralhealthradio.com/podcast/wahls

"Zach Wahls Speaks About Family." YouTube. Feb. 1, 2011. IowaHouseDemocrats. Accessed May 26, 2018. https://www.youtube.com/watch?v=FSQQK2Vuf9Q

Wolf, Robb. *The Paleo Solution: The Original Human Diet.* Las Vegas: Victory Belt. 2010.

Ballantyne, Sarah. The Paleo Approach: Reverse Autoimmune Disease and Heal Your Body. Victory Belt Publishing. 2014.

Davis, Dr. William. Jan. 16, 2017. "Grains: Perfect Obesogens." Wheat Belly blog. Accessed May 11, 2018. http://www.wheatbellyblog.com/2017/01/never-satisfied-maybe-not-fault/

Myss, Caroline. May 19, 2017. "Fact, Fiction, or Theory – Which Is Your Life?" Caroline's Blog. Accessed May 26, 2018. https://www.myss.com/fact-fiction-theory-life/

Yang, Qing. June 2010. "Gain weight by 'going diet?' Artificial sweeteners and the neurobiology of sugar cravings." Yale Journal of Biology and Medicine. Accessed April 19, 2018. https://www.ncbi.nlm.nih.gov/pmc/articles/PMC2892765/

Hari, Vani. Food Babe. Accessed May 26, 2018. https://foodbabe.com/

"Sugar: The Bitter Truth." YouTube. July 30, 2009. University of California Television (UCTV). Accessed Dec. 12, 2017. https://www.youtube.com/watch?v=dBnniua6-oM

Olney, John W., Farber, N. B., Spitznagel, E., Robins, L. N. November, 1996. "Increasing Brain Tumor Rates: Is There a Link to Aspartame?" Journal of Neuropathology & Experimental Neurology, Vol. 55, No. 11, pp. 1115-1123 doi: 10.1097/00005072-199611000-00002.

Romm, Aviva. Dec. 30, 2017. "Going with the Grain with Dr. Alan Christianson.".Aviva Romm MD Accessed May 26, 2018. https://avivaromm.com/alan-christianson/

Light therapy & sleep

National Sleep Foundation. 2013. "Obesity and Sleep." Accessed Feb. 12, 2018. https://sleepfoundation.org/sleep-topics/obesity-and-sleep/page/0/1

Mead, M. N. 2008. "Benefits of Sunlight: A Bright Spot for Human Health." Environmental Health Perspectives. 116(4):A160-A167. https://www.ncbi.nlm.nih.gov/pubmed/18414615

"Circadian Rhythms." August, 2107. National Institute of General Medical Sciences. Accessed May 23, 2018. https://www.nigms.nih.gov/Education/Pages/Factsheet_CircadianRhythms.aspx

Hansen, Fawne. Oct. 30, 2017. "How Do Cortisol Levels Change Throughout The Day?" Adrenal Fatigue Solution. Accessed March 26, 2018. https://adrenalfatiguesolution.com/cortisol-levels-change-throughout-day/

Duncan, Michael. April 25, 2017. "The Science of Wake-Up Lights, Sunrise Alarms, and Their Benefits." Be Right Light. Accessed May 26, 2018. https://www.berightlight.com/science-wake-lights-sunrise-alarms-benefits/

Adaptogens and other supplements

"Adaptogen Definition and Meaning | Collins English Dictionary." Complacent Definition and Meaning | Collins English Dictionary. Accessed June 14, 2018. https://www.collinsdictionary.com/dictionary/english/adaptogen.

Sargis, Dr. Robert M. April 2015. "An Overview of the Adrenal Glands." Endocrineweb. Accessed March 4, 2018. https://www.endocrineweb.com/endocrinology/overview-adrenal-glands

"Holy Basil: Overview, Uses, Side Effects, Interactions, Dosing." WebMD. Accessed May 26, 2018. https://www.webmd.com/vitamins/ai/ingredientmono-1101/holy-basil

Cohen, Marc M. 2014. "Tulsi: A Herb for all reasons." J-AIM. Journal of Ayurveda and Integrative Medicine. doi: 10.4103/0975-9476.146554. https://www.ncbi.nlm.nih.gov/pmc/articles/PMC4296439/Group, Dr. Edward F. Feb. 25, 2016. "Adaptogenic Herbs: What Are Adaptogens?" Global Healing Center. Accessed April 5, 2018. https://www.global healingcenter.com/natural-health/what-are-adaptogens/

Whelan, Richard. Lemon Balm. Richard Whelan Medical Herbalist. Accessed May 26, 2018. http://www.rjwhelan.co.nz/herbs A-Z/lemonbalm.html

Modi, M. B., Donga, S. B., Dei, L. October, 2012. "Clinical Evaluation of Ashokarishta, Ashwagandha Churna and Praval Pishti in the management of menopausal syndrome." International Quarterly Journal of Research in Ayurveda, Vol. 3, Issue 4, pp. 511-516. doi: 10.4103/0974-8520.110529. Accessed Jan.17, 2018. https://www.ncbi.nlm.nih.gov/pubmed/?term=Ashwaganda menopause

Anghelescu, I-G., Edwards, D., Seifritz, E., Kasper, S. (January, 2018) "Stress management and the role of Rhodiola rosea: a review." International Journal of Psychiatry in Clinical

Practice. doi: 10.1080/13651501.2017.1417442. https://www.ncbi.nlm.nih.gov/pubmed/29325481

Health Canada. March 22, 2012. "Vitamin D and Calcium: Updated Dietary Reference Intakes." Canada.ca. Accessed May 26, 2018. https://www.canada.ca/en/health-canada/services/food-nutrition/healthy-eating/vitamins-minerals/vitamin-calcium-updated-dietary-reference-intakes-nutrition.html

GrassrootsHealth. "Are you Vitamin D deficient?" Accessed Feb. 18, 2018. https://grassrootshealth.net/

Lam, Dr. Michael. 2016. "About GABA: An Ultimate Guide To Understanding This Neurotransmitter." Accessed April 6, 2018. https://www.drlam.com/blog/about-gaba/15864/

Exercise

Christianson, Alan. The Adrenal Reset Diet: Strategically Cycle Carbs and Proteins to Lose Weight, Balance Hormones, and Move from Stressed to Thriving. Harmony Books. 2014.

Levine, Dr. James A. August, 2014. "The Chairman's Curse: Lethal Sitting." Mayo Clinic Proceedings, Volume 89, Issue 8, pp. 1030-1032. Accessed May 10, 2018. https://www.mayoclinicproceedings.org/article/S0025-6196(14)00573-4/fulltext

Diaz, Keith M., Howard, V. J., Colabianchi, N., Vena, J. E., Safford, M. M., Blair, S. N., Hooker, S. P., Hutto, B. Oct. 03, 2017. "Patterns of Sedentary Behavior and Mortality in

U.S. Middle-Aged and Older Adults: A National Cohort Study." Annals of Internal Medicine. Accessed May 06, 2018. http://annals.org/aim/article-abstract/2653704/patterns-sed entary-behavior-mortality-u-s-middle-aged-older-adults

University of Leicester. Oct. 15, 2012. "New study finds that sitting for protracted periods increases the risk of diabetes, heart disease and death." Accessed May 06, 2018. https:// www2.le.ac.uk/offices/press/press-releases/2012/october/ new-study-finds-that-sitting-for-protracted-periods-increases-the-risk-of-diabetes-heart-disease-and-death

Boyles, Salynn. Oct.15, 2012. "Sitting Too Much May Lead to Diabetes, Heart Disease." WebMD. Accessed May 06, 2018. https://www.webmd.com/diabetes/news/20121015/ sitting-diabetes-heart-risks?src=RSS_PUBLIC

American Cancer Society. July 16, 2015. "Sitting Too Much Increases Cancer Risk in Women." Accessed May 06, 2018. https://www.cancer.org/latest-news/sitting-too-much-increas es-cancer-risk-in-women.html

Healy, Melissa. Jan. 19, 2015. "Even for the active, a long sit shortens life and erodes health." Los Angeles Times. Accessed May 06, 2018. http://www.latimes.com/science/sciencenow/ la-sci-sn-sitting-health-20150119-story.html

Duvivier, B. M. F. M., Schaper, N. C., Bremers, M. A., van Crombrugge, G., Menheere, P. P. C. A., Kars, M., Savelberg, H. C. M. Feb. 13, 2013. "Minimal Intensity Physical Activity (Standing and Walking) of Longer Duration Improves Insulin Action and Plasma Lipids More than Shorter Periods of Moderate to Vigorous Exercise (Cycling) in Sedentary Subjects When Energy Expenditure Is Comparable." PLOS Medicine. Accessed May 06, 2018. http://journals.plos.org/plosone/article?id=10.1371/journal.pone.0055542

Reducing your toxic load

World Health Organization. Feb. 1, 2018. "Cancer." Accessed April 8, 2018. http://www.who.int/news-room/fact-sheets/detail/cancer

Environmental Working Group. "About Us." EWG. Accessed April 8, 2018. https://www.ewg.org/about-us#.WwnYuC_MyiI

Environmental Working Group. "Clean Fifteen™ Conventional Produce with the Least Pesticides." EWG. Accessed Jan. 10, 2018. https://www.ewg.org/foodnews/clean-fifteen.php

BC Wolverton, B. C., Douglas, W. L., Bounds, K. July 1, 1989. "A Study of Indoor Landscape Plants for Indoor Air Pollution Abatement." Doc ID: 19930072988. https://ntrs.nasa.gov/search.jsp?R=19930072988

Chopra, Deepak. Super Genes: Unlock the Astonishing Power of Your DNA for Optimum Health and Well-Being. Random House UK. 2015.

Section 2: MIND - Header page

Norman Vincent Peale quote. Goodreads. Accessed Feb. 1, 2018. https://www.goodreads.com/quotes/33921-change-your-thoughts-and-you-change-your-world

Epiphany

"Epiphany." Dictionary.com. Accessed Feb. 1, 2018. http://www.dictionary.com/browse/epiphany

Sincero, Jen. You Are a Badass: How to stop doubting your greatness and start living an awesome life. Running Press. 2013.

Harris, Dan. 10% Happier: How I Tamed the Voice in My Head, Reduced Stress without Losing My Edge, and Found Self-help That Actually Works – A True Story. London, England: Yellow Kite. 2017.

Command your body

Hansen, Fawne. Oct. 30, 2017. "How Do Cortisol Levels Change Throughout The Day?" Adrenal Fatigue Solution. Accessed March 26, 2018. https://adrenalfatiguesolution.com/cortisol-levels-change-throughout-day/

Wounds of the helper

Child Welfare Information Gateway. 2015. "Understanding the effects of maltreatment on brain development. U.S. Department of Health and Human Services, Children's Bureau. https://www.childwelfare.gov/pubs/issue-briefs/brain-development/

Myss, Caroline. *Why People Don't Heal and How They Can.* Three Rivers Press. 1997.

Van Vlack, Tasha. Nov. 3, 2017. "Warning Signs of Vicarious Trauma/Secondary Traumatic Stress and Compassion Fatigue." TEND®. Accessed May 26, 2018. http://www.tendacademy.ca/warning-signs-of-vicarious-traumasecondary-traumatic-stress-and-compassion-fatigue/

Center For Substance Abuse Treatment. Jan. 1, 1970. "Substance Abuse Treatment for Persons with Child Abuse and Neglect Issues." Chapter 4 – "Therapeutic Issues for Counselors." Accessed March 27, 2018. https://www.ncbi.nlm.nih.gov/books/NBK64902/

Self-Talk and internal dialogue

Myss, Caroline. "Take Charge of Your Health." Myss.com. Accessed May 26, 2018. https://www.myss.com/free-resources/take-charge/take-charge-of-your-health/

Ellis, Albert. "Rational Psychotherapy and Individual Psychology." All-about-psychology.com. Accessed May 26,

2018. https://www.all-about-psychology.com/rational-psy chotherapy.html

Halvorson, Heidi Grant. March 14, 2013. "The Amazing Power of 'I Don't' vs. 'I Can't'." Forbes. Accessed May 27, 2018. https://www.forbes.com/sites/heidigranthalvorson/2013/03/14/the-amazing-power-of-i-dont-vs-i-cant/#7455f990d037

Greatness

Warren Buffett Quote. Brainy Quote. Accessed May 26, 2018. https://www.brainyquote.com/quotes/warren_buffett_409214

Suzuki, David. June 1, 2017. "World Environment Day Reminds Us to Reconnect with Nature." David Suzuki Foundation. Accessed May 26, 2018. https://davidsuzuki.org/story/world-environment-day-reminds-us-reconnect-nature/

The great unveiling

Alan Cohen Quote. Quotefancy. https://quotefancy.com/quote/761166/Alan-Cohen-The-purpose-of-life-is-not-to-fight-against-evil-and-misfortune-it-is-to Nikola Tesla Quote. "The Motors I Build There Were Exactly as I Imagined Them. I Made No Attempt to Improve the Design, but Merely Reproduced..." (12 Wallpapers) - Quotefancy. Accessed May 26, 2018. https://quotefancy.com/quote/876566/Nikola-Tesla-The-motors-I-build-there-were-exactly-as-I-imagined-them-I-made-no-attempt

Releasing fear

Selig, Paul. *The Book of Truth: A Channeled Text*. Tarcher Perigee. 2017.

Sincero, Jen. You Are a Badass: How to stop doubting your greatness and start living an awesome life. Running Press. 2013.

Sherman, Jeremy E. April 17, 2014. "Psychological Crutches: Ten Myths and Three Tips." Psychology Today. Accessed April 18, 2018. https://www.psychologytoday.com/us/blog/ambigamy/201404/psychological-crutches-ten-myths-and-three-tips

Possibility

Audrey Hepburn quote. Beed media. http://www.beedmedia.com/motivational-quotes/nothing-is-impossible-the-word-itself-says-i-m-possible-andrey-hepburn/andrey-hepburn/

Unknown quote. Tiny Buddha. Accessed May 26, 2018. https://tinybuddha.com/wisdom-quotes/don-t-fear-failure-so-much-that-you-refuse-to-try-new-things-the-saddest-summary-of-life-contains-three-descriptions-could-have-might-have-and-should-have/

Section 3: SPIRIT - What is spirituality

"Spiritual." English Oxford Living Dictionaries. Accessed May 26, 2018. https://en.oxforddictionaries. com/definition/spiritual

"Existential Crisis." Wikipedia. Accessed May 26, 2018. https://en.wikipedia.org/wiki/Existential_crisis

Challenging your agreements

Selig, Paul. *The Book of Truth: A Channeled Text*. Tarcher Perigee. 2017.

A beacon of truth

Selig, Paul. *The Book of Truth: A Channeled Text*. Tarcher Perigee. 2017.

Albert, Jim, and Herbert, Margot. 2006. "Child Welfare." The Canadian Encyclopedia. Accessed May 26, 2018. http://www.thecanadianencyclopedia.ca/en/article/child-welfare/

Perspective is everything

"Yanny." May 2018. Wikipedia. Accessed May 27, 2018. https://en.wikipedia.org/wiki/Yanny_or_Laurel

"Cognitive dissonance.", Wikipedia. Accessed May 7, 2018. https://en.wikipedia.org/w/index.php?title=Cognitive_dissonance&oldid=839617204

Gratitude

David Steindl-Rast quote. Goodreads. Accessed May 27, 2018. https://www.goodreads.com/author/quotes/4182.David_Steindl_Rast

Tolle, Eckhart. The Power of NOW: A Guide to Spiritual Enlightenment. Namaste Publishing. 2004

Forgiveness

Oprah Winfrey quote. PassItOn.com. Accessed May 27, 2018. https://www.passiton.com/inspirational-quotes/7394-true-forgiveness-is-when-you-can-say-thank

Podrazik, Joan. March 11, 2013. "Oprah on forgiveness: This definition was 'bigger than an aha moment'." Huffington Post. Accessed May 27, 2018. https://www.huffingtonpost.com/2013/03/07/oprah-on-forgiveness-how-to-forgive_n_2821736.html

Generosity

Aesop quote. Wikiquote. Accessed May 27, 2018. https://en.wikiquote.org/wiki/Aesop

Myss, Caroline. Invisible Acts of Power: Personal Choices That Create Miracles. London: Pocket. 2007.

Audrey Hepburn quote. PassItOn.com. Accessed May 27, 2018. https://www.passiton.com/inspirational-quotes/6596-as-you-grow-older-you-will-discover-that-you

Mindfulness & meditation

James Baraz quote. Goodreads. Accessed May 27, 2018. https://www.goodreads.com/quotes/232890-mindfulness-is-simply-being-aware-of-what-is-happening-right

Thich Nhat Hanh quote. The Art of Power. Goodreads. Accessed May 27, 2018. https://www.goodreads.com/quotes/142660-to-dwell-in-the-here-and-now-does-not-mean

Boyd, Lara. December 15, 2015. "After watching this, your brain will not be the same." TEDx Vancouver. YouTube. Accessed May 27, 2018. https://www.youtube.com/watch?v=LNHBMFCzznE&vl=en

Miklowitz, David J., Alatiq, Y., Goodwin, G. M., Geddes, J. R., Fennell, M. J. V., Dimidjian, S., Hauser, M., Williams, J. M. G. 2009. "A Pilot Study of Mindfulness-based Cognitive Therapy for Bipolar Disorder." International Journal of Cognitive Therapy. Vol. 2, Issue 4, pp. 373-382 https://guilfordjournals.com/doi/10.1521/ijct.2009.2.4.373

Hölzel, B. K., Carmody, J., Vangel, M., Congleton, C., Yerramsetti, S. M., Gard, T., & Lazar, S. W. (2011).

Mindfulness practice leads to increases in regional brain gray matter density. *Psychiatry Research, 191*(1), 36–43. http://doi.org/10.1016/j.pscychresns.2010.08.006

"Start Here! 5 Meditation Styles for Beginners." The Chopra Center. February 11, 2017. Accessed June 24, 2018. https://chopra.com/articles/start-here-5-meditation-styles-for-beginners.

"Mantra's." Finding Your Happiness. August 08, 2016. Accessed June 24, 2018. https://createbalanceandfindinghappiness.wordpress.com/2016/08/08/mantras/.

Worth

Kaplan, Connie. The Invisible Garment: 30 Spiritual Principles That Weave the Fabric of Human Life. Jodere Group. 2004.

Higher purpose

Joseph Campbell quote. Brainy quote. Accessed May 27, 2018. https://www.brainyquote.com/quotes/joseph_campbell_138795

Self-love

Ralph Waldo Emerson quote. Wattpad, Quotable Quotes: Book II. Accessed May 27, 2018. https://www.wattpad.com/41462157-quotable-quotes-book-ii-what-lies-inside-you

Louise Hay Quote. Brainy Quote. Accessed May 27, 2018. https://www.brainyquote.com/quotes/louise_l_hay_178047

Practice makes perfect

Bruce Lee quote. Luke Rockhold, MMA-Core.com Accessed May 27, 2018. https://www.mma-core.com/photos/Luke_Rockhold_IG_Post_I_fear_not_the_man_who_has_prac ticed_10_000_kicks_once_but_I_fear_the_man_who_has_practiced/182035

Desmond Tutu quote. Propeller. Accessed May 27, 2018. https://www.propeller.la/tutu4

Other sources

Myss, Caroline. Invisible Acts of Power: The Divine Energy of a Giving Heart. London: Pocket. 2007.

Dalai Lama; Tutu, Desmond; Abrams, Douglas Carlton. The Book of Joy. Penguin Canada. 2016.

Bishop, Gary John. Unfu*k Yourself: Get out of Your Head and into Your Life. Harper One. 2017.

About the author

I live in the diverse suburb of Mississauga, Ontario. I am the wife of a supportive and loving person, Karen Bruer, since October of 2007. Seemingly, many of my "titles" begin with the word mom. I am a dance mom, a twin mom, a step-mom of 3, and a retired treatment foster parent after 18 years of active service. I am a Child and Youth Counsellor. I am an unapologetic feminist lesbian. My hobbies include scrapbooking, weight lifting, hiking, biking, yoga and all things mindfulness related.

I want the world to know how undervalued helpers have been. I want the community to know that they have left helpers high-and-dry buried in a cycle of mental health, child abuse, poverty and pain. I want the world to stop sweeping all of it under the rug.

Social service communities need more funding, more resources, more innovation. Our world need to place more value on its helpers.

We need to implement self-care and burnout strategies for our helpers and show tenderness toward the pain that comes with these various professions. We need to acknowledge how much "policy" can damage the system of helping, we need a policy for eye contact, we need a policy for permission to access our gut feelings.

When a school shooting happens, I want the world to acknowledge that placing *helpers* at the bottom is a real smoking gun.

Artistic contribution

ANGELA LIPSCOMBE CZT

The inspiring painting on the front cover is called "Trillium Forest" which is thanks to Angela Lipscombe of Ontario, Canada, she also provided the small tiles of Zentangle© on the back cover, thanks so much Angela for your artistic contribution.

A native of Port Credit, Ontario, Angela Lipscombe is an award winning Visual Artist, Art Instructor, Graphic Designer and Certified Zentangle® Teacher (CZT) where her career and accomplishments span over 35 years. Angela's primary focus now is on teaching the love of art in all mediums to children, youth, adults and seniors in her home studio of Oakville, the Milton Centre for the Arts, and to various public and private art organizations. Angela's work can be found at various art exhibitions throughout the year and on her website drawntoart.ca.

43406048R00126

Made in the USA
Middletown, DE
23 April 2019